RECLAIMING YOU

The Simple Wellness Guide for Health and Happiness for Over 45s

Jeanette Herrington

First published by Ultimate World Publishing 2020
Copyright © 2020 Jeanette Herrington

ISBN

Paperback: 978-1-922497-06-2
Ebook: 978-1-922497-07-9

Cover design: Ultimate World Publishing
Layout and typesetting: Ultimate World Publishing
Editor: Marinda Wilkinson
Cover photographer: Peter Herrington
Illustrations: Pamela Carrington

Ultimate World Publishing
Diamond Creek,
Victoria Australia 3089
www.writeabook.com.au

ULTIMATE WORLD
PUBLISHING

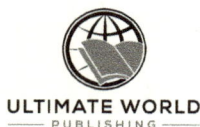

Disclaimer

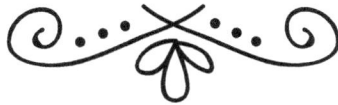

This book aims to provide readers with inspiration and information, but it is not intended to be a substitute for personal, health or medical advice from a qualified professional. Always seek the guidance of your doctor or other qualified health professional with any questions you may have regarding your health or a medical condition. The author and publisher claim no responsibility to any person for any liability, loss or damage caused or alleged to be caused directly or indirectly as a result of the use, application or interpretation of the material in this book.

Testimonials

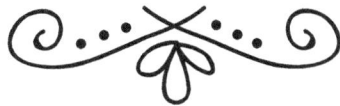

'I met Jeanette over 20 years ago when we were both horse riding together. Fast-forward about 10 years and through circumstances we reconnected. I discovered Jeanette had become a personal trainer and decided to have some sessions with her. Wow, I was newly into triathlon then, and Jeanette was able to program my sessions to help me in my new sport. She also made the sessions so much fun, and I never knew what we were going to do week to week. I loved how she made me feel, and because of this, I decided to embark on a new career as a personal trainer myself. I have now been in the fitness industry for seven years and love it. Thank you, Jeanette, for everything you've done and inspired me to be.'

Sue, personal trainer

'Jeanette is a very caring and perceptive person, and her gentle and encouraging manner always made me feel at ease. I have learned so much in her classes, not just from the basic exercises that we all know but from the little tweaks that make them so much more effective.'

Chris, Roll Back the Clock participant

'I have worked with Jeanette primarily after my pregnancies to ease myself back into fitness. She showed me how to do the exercises safely while building up my stamina. She introduced me to the TRX, and I absolutely loved this kind of new equipment to work with. She is such a lovely, caring person who was interested in my life and my journey in the gym. She always prepared well for our session and pushed me when I needed a push (no whingeing was allowed) and slowed me down when I went too crazy. I absolutely loved working with her!'

Desirée, 41 years

'Jeanette was a wonderful person to work with as a personal trainer. She is extremely caring and considerate, making sure that my workout was suitable for my capabilities but at the same time pushing me to the limit she knew I could achieve. I loved working with Jeanette as she was so friendly and happy every day.'

Di M, personal training client

'I started training with Jeanette after a long time away from the gym following an ongoing injury. It was quite daunting stepping back into the gym, but Jeanette eased the way with tailored workouts that worked with my injury while challenging and improving my overall strength and fitness. Jeanette's workouts are fun and varied and I particularly enjoy our outdoor boxing sessions! Jeanette is always positive, enthusiastic and encouraging. She takes the time to listen and demonstrates the equipment and movements to make sure that the exercise is safe and effective. My confidence with strength exercises has improved greatly since working with Jeanette and I have achieved my goal to lift weights in the gym!'

Amanda, 49 years

'I had suffered a series of health issues which meant I could no longer keep up my previous exercise routine. I was worried about being socially isolated and found out about "Roll Back the Clock". It was just what I wanted. Jeanette's friendly approach to fitness was all inclusive and made me feel more motivated. Everyone was treated equally, and I wasn't alone anymore. I can't wait for the sessions to start again.'

Jane, Roll Back the Clock participant

'Just wanted to say that I thought you were lovely with our bowls group ... exuberant but very mindful of our abilities and ages. I enjoyed attending your sessions. Thanks.'

Leonie, Roll Back the Clock participant

Dedication

♥

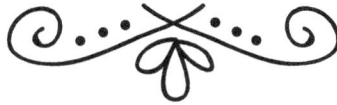

For my parents, Pamela and Malcolm, for giving me a happy, healthy upbringing with plenty of love and laughter in an idyllic country setting. I'm so very, very grateful.

Your positive role modelling has inspired me throughout life and in my own wellness journey.

And for my beautiful daughters, Charlize and Amberley, you motivate me to stay on track with my health and I'm so proud to be your mum! Thank you for the love, fun and joy you bring to my life. xx

Reclaiming You

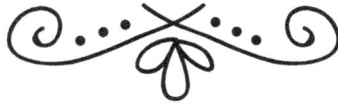

I'm on a quest to learn
how I can energise,
to find my life's true purpose
and now I'll fantasise …

I want to delve deeper
to discover my own big *Why*,
and dream about my future
wishing that I could fly.

To soar amongst the clouds
and be free of any fear,
light and energetic
feeling joy and full of cheer.

Sparked by my vision
showing me the way,
fuelled by a passion
in case that I should stray.

My healthy goals and habits
focused and in sight,
aligned with my vision
by a beam of guiding light.

What a wonderful adventure
feeling better every day,
loving my healthy body
with new habits here to stay.

Wellness is a privilege!
To feel a sense of new!
Be patient on this journey …
and enjoy *Reclaiming You*!

By Jeanette Herrington

Contents

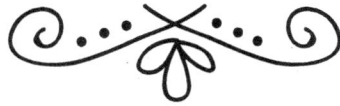

Introduction

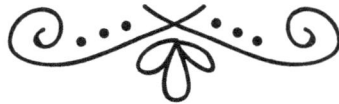

WHO WANTS A QUICK FIX?

There are times when we all secretly wish for a **quick-fix** solution! Realistically though, we know we need more than a 12-week body blitz special at the local gym to do the trick, if we want results that last.

I've certainly wished I could wave my magic wand and conjure up an instant fix. I've had clients wanting that too, as they re-enrolled optimistically year after year, for their annual 'body blitz' fix.

After the 12-week program, they would parade their fab new bodies, success banners flying high. But what happened afterwards? Was that 'quick fix' all it was cracked up to be? It was for some, who used the springtime 'extra', to reinvigorate and nudge them back onto the path. *Brilliant.* But did you notice I said, *some*?

What happened to the rest of the gang?

They soldiered on for a short while, then disappeared one by one, going back to their old pre-blitz habits … until next year, when they returned ready to do it all over again. While always keen to help them get back on track, I was curious about how I could also help them during those other nine months outside of the program. What did they need to stay motivated and keep their new healthy habits going? Not all could keep up the cost and commitment of personal training. I wanted them to use the annual blitz as a fun, springtime detox, instead of the huge overhaul they required, year after year with disappointment in between.

Had I failed them, and not provided enough education or skills to see them through? I searched for answers and experimented on clients who were prepared to be my guinea pigs. I discovered that a shift in mindset and good foundations were vital at the **beginning** of their journey. Whilst the springtime booster had value and fun, without that strong foundation, the results just didn't last.

Strong foundations are important, like any builder will tell you. And in health and fitness, uncovering your big 'why' reasons at the start of the process, is what will inspire you to continue on the journey for **life**.

It's true that your wellness journey may be challenging at times—but it will also be rewarding, filled with enjoyment and give you a deep sense of satisfaction. Not to mention the myriad of amazing benefits that good health brings to every aspect of your life.

What will you learn in this book?

Throughout this book you will learn skills, tools and strategies to kickstart your journey towards better health. Whether you are part of the annual blitz team or starting from scratch, you will discover how to enjoy the journey from year to year forever, not just in sporadic bursts. You will learn how to find your inner spark to fire up and sustain you when you need an extra pick-me-up and explore why the foundational steps are so important. I will walk you through, one step at a time, so you feel confident and supported in moving forward and getting the results you want and more.

Your experience will be unique, just like you. One size does not fit all. I had wondered why a certain exercise program or diet may work for eight out of ten people, but not the other two who followed the plan religiously. When they didn't get the results they had expected, despite doing everything they had been asked, their confidence was sapped. It was demoralising for them and I wanted to help. I heard about a new ground-breaking personalised health platform based around the science of epigenetics. I felt this could be the missing piece of the puzzle, and I am currently completing further studies to help clients reach their own personal potential using this platform. So, in the spirit of knowing we are all unique, I won't be preaching in this book on what foods or specific exercises are best for you. I do offer advice in these areas, but it is of general information only, to be used as a starting point for you to explore further.

Whet your appetite with exercise

This book will also inspire you to explore new options around physical activity. Do YOU like the gym? I was once terrified to walk into a gym on my own, so I didn't. For many years I avoided it, secretly wishing I belonged to the cool crowd who knew what they were doing, calmly and confidently. If this is you, then I will hold your hand and demystify that scary jungle. If you already have a regular fitness plan, I will encourage you to step outside your comfort zone to ensure you keep fresh and challenged.

Who is the book for?

Ageing is inevitable and comes with a host of changes in your body and brain. This book is aimed at women over the age of 45 however the value is there for everyone: young or old, even the men! **Why 45?**

Here are a few good reasons:

- It is an age when women (or men) can often hit a wall. Health that has previously been taken for granted, can now start to show cracks. It was the age for me, when I first encountered difficulties that previously I'd managed so well.

- Research shows that chronic diseases feature more prominently among people **aged 45 and over**.

- Being fit and healthy can help to manage hormonal symptoms. If this doesn't apply to you now, keep it in mind for the future. If you are already in the midst or on the other side of menopause, exercise can be a great outlet, particularly for those with fiery volcanos erupting!

A little more about me…

I start this book by sharing my story of who I was 15 years ago, when I was aged 45. At that time, I battled to regain my fitness and energy after struggling with the competing demands of motherhood. I felt exhausted, with a lack of confidence on where to begin. As you will see, I did get back on track and have maintained my fitness—and I want to help others who are struggling to do the same.

I have been a fitness professional now for 12 years. In this book I reflect on my clients' stories, changing some names and circumstances to protect their identity. I'm so grateful for everything I have learned from them. Thank you for trusting me and allowing me to share your stories as well as teaching me more about myself, and how to assist others.

On reflection, if I'd been able to fast-track the process with a quick zap of the wand, I may have missed out on the incredible learning experiences I've had. My own personal wellness and professional journey has had its fair share of ups and downs along the way, and I embrace those as learning opportunities to grow strength and wisdom. I plan to continue on in my quest to grow a little wiser and stronger every day.

Writing this book has been a wonderful experience and I'm so proud to share it with you. My goal is to help you increase your personal awareness; to empower you to seek out answers, become your own expert and bring about lasting positive changes to your health. I want to encourage you to incorporate healthy behaviours into your everyday life and do so from a position of positivity, not beat yourself up because you feel you 'have to'. I want you to experience the joy of exercise and associate it with happiness and feel-good endorphins as you explore how to best achieve great energy, good health and wellness.

This book does not aim to compete with the thousands of other wellness books on the market. This is my own unique guide to getting back on track, based on personal experience and that of my clients. I hope you will find me to be a relatable companion; someone that's walked in your shoes.

Please enjoy reading RECLAIMING YOU!

CHAPTER 1

Up Close and Personal
Your call to action

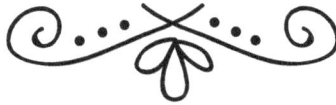

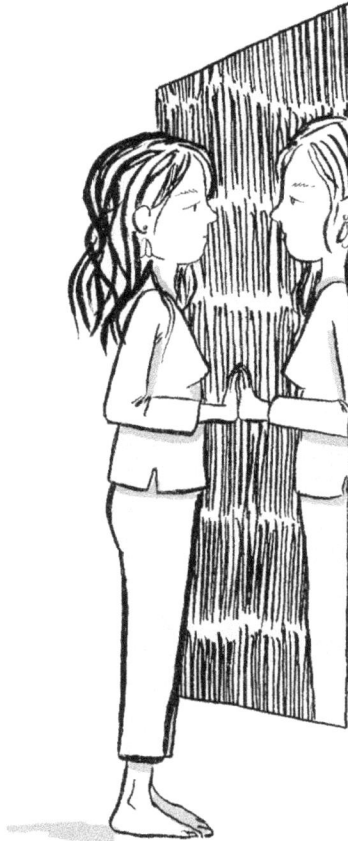

'I don't want other people to decide who I am.
I want to decide that for myself.'

– Emma Watson

'*How old are your grandkids?*' I had been asked a simple, innocent question but the effect on me was profound. It hit a raw nerve and prompted a plethora of emotions to surface.

Have you ever put off taking action that you knew would be good for you, but delayed it day after day? Perhaps you wanted to start a new health regime and the timing to start was never quite right, and you brushed it over it with thoughts like *I'll wait until after Christmas, Monday sounds good, Dry July is coming up soon ...*

Hindsight is a wonderful thing and it had me wondering what finally prompts us into taking action that we know will be good for us. What helps us reach that point of, *I'm not going to take this another minute longer?*

Emotions can reveal what matters to us and what doesn't. They can shine light on a situation to help us, and there are lessons to be learned IF we are receptive and ready to use them to embrace change and propel us into action. This can be difficult when we experience uncomfortable emotions, and it can be tempting to bury them or cast them aside with busyness and distraction techniques. Sometimes, we hurriedly pop them away in the filing cabinet, in folders suggestive of procrastination or excuses, as we tell ourselves that we will deal with it on *another day* when the planets are all lined up. That 'day' could be tomorrow, but it also might be a long time coming—or never arrive.

If we can look at those uncomfortable feelings squarely in the face and bring them out into the daylight, we have the choice and potential to use them as our very own *call to action*. It doesn't mean we will suddenly stop feeling uncomfortable and be presented with a platter full of solutions. There is definitely some work to be done. But the positive benefits can be life-changing! We can jump back into the driver's seat to explore new possibilities, through fresh eyes, to take back ownership and *then* decide on the best way forward.

My call to action came in the form of those five small words. Almost 15 years ago now, I was a 45-year-old 'older mum' with two daughters aged 10 months and two. The 'grandma' question came from a beautician who I'd gone to see for a waxing appointment.

*Flustered from rushing and seriously out of breath from pushing the heavy double pram, I arrived at the shops for my appointment. After hearing the question, I was taken aback and almost embarrassed to say that they were, in fact, my **children**, NOT my grandchildren!*

I waited expectedly for her to backtrack like, 'Oh sorry, it's not that you LOOK like their grandmother'. She COULD lie. After all, I was a new client! She hesitated with a surprised expression and eyebrow lift and dismissed my answer. 'Ohhhh! Well come on through and let's get those eyebrows waxed'. I tried to pretend it didn't bother me and I certainly didn't want to appear angry with her. After all, she might take revenge and wax off my whole eyebrows!

It was a fair enough assumption because I was technically old enough to be a grandma, but it triggered something inside of me. I felt hurt and couldn't wait to get home. With twice the amount of huff and puff, I pushed the pram at a lightning pace so I could put the girls down for a lunchtime sleep and scrutinise myself in the mirror.

I considered my options: Do I bury my hurt under the rug and go about business as usual? Whinge to someone? Tempting. I knew I could count on a sympathetic friend to say, 'How DARE she!'. But why should I care what a total stranger thought? And is that what others saw too? After deep consideration, I realised that I felt upset because it brought to the surface, emotions of 'I don't feel good about myself'. I decided to take a closer look. Bring on the mirror ...

Looking back now, the actual trigger event was quite insignificant. Yet, the emotions raised were powerful, and caused me to take action that I had been procrastinating about for months.

'You can't change what you don't acknowledge.'
– Dr Phil, Psychologist and Television Host

This quote resonated with me and I'd heard it from Dr Phil many times. Watching Oprah and Dr Phil was a lunchtime indulgence when the girls had their nap. There is so much truth in that phrase. It really means looking at your life and taking responsibility for it. Truly owning it. If you can acknowledge your situation and bring awareness to your feelings, then this will open the door to conscious choice and the possibilities beyond.

Mirror audit

The girls were sleeping peacefully, and I decided to skip the lunchtime combo of Dr Phil paired with domestic chores in the ad breaks.

It was the moment of truth. I went into full-blown 'acknowledgement' with a comprehensive critique of my grandma status. I started with the obvious … well my freshly waxed eyebrows were great. Good start! Mmmmmm, I went into dissection mode and checked out wrinkles, teeth, eyes (slightly red and puffy). After a full-blown audit of my hair, face and body (the girls slept long that day), I came up with a list of things that I wasn't happy about:

- *Out of breath just from wheeling the pram and light housework (**unfit**)*
- *Rounded posture from 'mum' duties (**weak postural muscles**)*
- *Puffy eyes from lack of sleep (**tired**)*

4

- *Smile okay, but was it reaching my eyes or was it one of those autopilot 'yes, I'm fine thanks, how are you?' sort of smiles* **(unhappy about self)**
- *Body, too heavy by around 20kg but was too scared to hop on the scales! I was exhausted. My knees were suffering from the overloaded stress* **(overweight and muscle weakness)**
- *Clothing felt undesirable on so many levels. I had a love/hate relationship with my frumpy elasticated clothes. They were comfy, but so are trackies* **(unhappy with baggy clothing).**

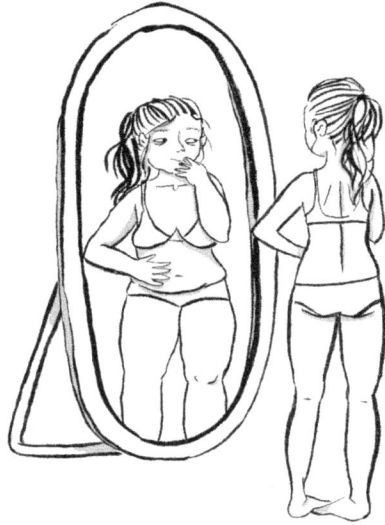

*Indulging in some rare vanity, those were some of the physical things I saw and felt. I tried to retain some perspective and reassure myself that they were merely temporary physical things that I could address if I really tried. More importantly though, was the way I **felt** with a range of emotions that had me feeling miserable. If I addressed the physical things, would I feel happier and just how long had I felt that way?*

*I guess those feelings were there every day—like an annoying, nagging, fleeting thought that got pushed to the side and ignored, whilst thinking 'one day I've got to fix that'. I really wanted to get rid of the baggy, hide-all clothing, but at some level had been telling myself that it wasn't the right time. A little alarm was now going off in my head chanting 'Excuses!' When **would** the right time be and why wasn't I doing it now?*

There were also some feelings of guilt to explore. Did I have the right to be unhappy about my appearance when I had just achieved my lifelong dream of having two adorable, healthy daughters with a supportive husband?

5

I did feel enormous gratitude for many things, including my beautiful family. I concluded that if I could take back the reins to improve my overall health, then surely it would restore my confidence and happiness, and we would all benefit. With the saying in mind about **'putting your own oxygen mask on first'**, *I made the decision to take back ownership to restore my health and be the happy, confident, energetic person that I knew I was capable of being.*

Thank you, Waxing Lady, (even though at the time, I was still furious at her insensitivity!). I wasn't going to spend another precious moment living under a veil of excuses with time slipping away. It was time to own it and go for it with no blame on anyone else. I was ready to grab that steering wheel and find a way to make it happen. Now ... what to do and where to start?

Actually, I had *already* started just by facing up to the truth and realising I had choices, and it was now up to me. If you have any discontent around your own health, fitness, nutrition or mindset, whether it is a slight niggle simmering below the surface or is collecting dust in your procrastination or excuses folder, this is what I encourage you to do too.

To move forward, exploring wellness and reclaiming your happiness and zest for life, must start with bringing awareness to your body and mind and making a commitment to change. I've broken this down into a three-step guide:

1. BRING AWARENESS TO YOUR HEALTH

Who do YOU think you are? Getting up close and personal

Think about your current state of health. Remember, this is YOUR journey and is not about making changes to please anyone else. Do you feel energised and vibrant? What areas of your health would you like to improve?

When our bodies are out of sync, symptoms can develop over time such as low energy, fatigue, stress, aches and pains. They are our body's way of signalling that we need to pay attention! If we take heed and become more aware of what our bodies need, we can focus our attention in the right area to restore optimal health.

Some of you may have a list like mine. Others may love the person they see in the mirror and want to make some minor tweaks or become more physically fit. We are all at different stages and need to identify any health aspect that requires our attention to create new behaviours around.

This is also a great opportunity to focus on yourself to develop new strategies for the future, and to check that your toolbox of 'just in case' tips and tricks is fresh and up to date. Just as the COVID-19 pandemic changed the lives of everyone, we don't know what is around the corner, so it makes sense to have a strong immune system and your toolbox filled with useful strategies.

If you don't take time out now to focus consciously on your health, you may become complacent and your situation routine or stagnant— or you might become ill, or even worse!

Up close and personal exercise

Use this opportunity now to be totally focused on yourself ...

- Face the mirror (or not) and assume full responsibility without negativity. **If you're game enough strip down and have a real good look!** Treat yourself with compassion and commit to being your own best friend.

7

- Jot down a list of any health issues, desired outcomes or goals you would like to address and how they make you feel. It may be that you feel tired or unfit, or you would like to lose weight. Your list can be as long and exhaustive as you feel it has to be. It doesn't mean you need to work on everything on that list right now. Keep in mind, that one super remedy may improve lots of issues at once. For example, an increase in physical exercise can resolve MANY complaints. Likewise, improving your nutrition and mind health can too.
- Take note of any stiffness, aches or pains that could be managed better. Is there more you could do to manage a physical injury? Are you a healthy weight that feels right for you? Carrying extra weight can make you feel tired and sluggish.
- Are you happy with your sleep habits? Do you manage stress effectively? Are you shallow breathing and rushing around to achieve as much as you can?

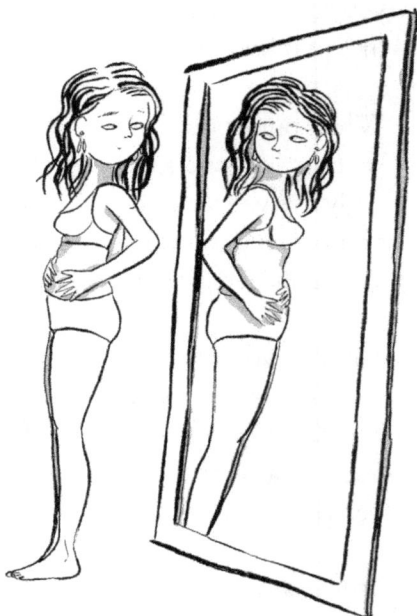

Bear in mind that it is not about what you feel you *should* look like. You can be overweight in the eyes of society, but it's all about how you feel inside: your own perception. I can recall how I felt at that mirror audit time, and yet, when I looked for some photos recently, I saw myself in a totally different light. My disguise and emotional mask were effective! Only *you* know how you feel, and this book is about *you and RECLAIMING YOU!*

After bringing awareness to how you feel, it's time to consider change and how to get started. If you are ready to pull back the blinds and get moving with change, then a commitment is required. I find the people that invest time to lay good foundations, become more in touch with their feelings and emotions, which leads to a greater and longer-lasting transformation.

2. COMMITMENT TO CHANGE

Change can be scary and means stepping out of our comfort zones and into the unknown. Our brain wants to keep us safe, and we sometimes need to push ourselves into the *uncomfortable,* to achieve success in unchartered territories. You may need some extra support or guidance with this. When we lack confidence around knowing what our capabilities are, putting trust in an adviser can help us to see the possibilities for ourselves, whilst we learn and develop more trust in our own judgement.

If you don't have the right support, you might go back to your comfort zone, putting plans on hold, again. **Are you ready to make a commitment to change?**

I use a visualisation technique with clients before we embark on the fitness side of things. It can bring that sense of urgency that we don't want to waste more time just *talking* about what we *know* we want to do.

Visualisations

Before doing this exercise, think back to those areas of health that you desire to change, with an emphasis on your feelings around this. With this focus in mind, you will imagine your future.

Find a place with no distractions where you can travel forward in your mind to a time period of six months or a year from now. I generally suggest 12 months because it can be easier to picture yourself on the same date or month by association with an annual event, for example, a birthday.

I recommend that you close your eyes to assist in making this visualisation as real as possible and perhaps have someone help you with the exercise.

Tailor the words to fit your own situation and I'll talk you through an example.

Visualisation 1:
Visualise it is 12 months from today and you are sitting in the same place as you are now, your situation unchanged. You had intended to be feeling much healthier and happier. You had tried to introduce new behaviours around {tailor wording for your situation}. Perhaps you started off really well a year ago, but after a few weeks, you hit a roadblock. Something happened and it got hard to keep up the motivation. Imagine how you feel, one year on. Your situation has stayed the same ...

Ask yourself: What's happening in your life? How does your body feel? How do you feel in your mind? Is the problem the same or worse? If you had this one year over again, what would you do differently? What are you feeling if you knew what to do and didn't do it?

Pause and reflect on your feelings before doing Visualisation 2.

If I had looked ahead 12 months and had not made changes to my health, my visualisation would have been something like this:
The ongoing struggle of tiredness and heaviness, hauling myself up from the floor by holding onto the couch, being puffed out as I tried to keep up with

my two active girls. I was still cringing about what to wear when invited out and sticking to black, minimising clothing. I hated opening up the wardrobe scouring for something to wear that felt and looked good. I had some anger that 12 months had gone past and I was still in the same position, only it was worse because the girls were a year older and even more active. I was still struggling to keep up with the busy demands of motherhood ... I felt disappointed and unhappy for letting myself and my family down.

Visualisation 2:

I want you to visualise what you will be doing and how you feel in 12 months if today is a fresh new start. You've decided to grab hold of this opportunity and make a commitment to do what it takes to get on the path to RECLAIM YOU and feel your absolute best! It's one year on and you have nailed it and developed new sustainable habits by practising behaviours that make it easier every day to stay on the path. You are blitzing your health goals.

Ask yourself: What's happening in your life? What's changed? How does your body feel? How do you feel in your mind? How confident do you feel? Proud? Happy?

My second visualisation would have looked like this:

Yep, I could still be mistaken for a grandma, but it would be like water off a duck's back—who cares what anyone thinks! I had some sass and attitude or perhaps it was confidence. I had so much energy to play with my kids. The only huffing and puffing would be intentional ... marathons (no not really), exercise classes with new friends and other fun, sexy reasons. I would be wearing my fitted hot pink coloured sporty gear as all the baggy frumpy stuff was gone. I'd be at the shops strutting past the beauticians, with a spring in my step coz I didn't have to carry that extra 20kg around! I'd give the beautician a cheeky wave with a big genuine beaming smile and inwardly thank her for prompting me to examine what was lurking beneath and allowing my true feelings to rise to the surface. I was feeling proud and happy that I had introduced changes to feel better.

11

These visualisations can significantly improve your level of commitment and my clients often report feeling relieved and happy that it was only an exercise. Some have said they felt like they were given a second chance, a gift of time with *Phew, lucky I've now got the choice of how I want to spend the next year!* However, just a word of warning. This exercise can be confronting for some. It can bring further emotions to the surface that can be even more uncomfortable. Please reach out for support if you need additional help. We all respond differently, as I'll demonstrate with Cynthia's experience, a 52-year-old high school teacher.

Cynthia's story

Cynthia had been battling with menopausal symptoms, had gained extra weight and was feeling frumpy and unhappy. She was not enjoying teaching because she was snappy and irritable. Her doctor had suggested that some changes to her diet and regular exercise would help and also be a good outlet for stress and assist in levelling out the hormones. She was embarrassed to go back to her doctor and admit to not taking the recommended advice.

Cynthia's body language was defeatist. She was drained, sick and tired of feeling out of sorts. This was the perfect student, ready to do whatever I suggested. I didn't want this to be a one-hit wonder with a quick burst of personal training designed to lose weight. I really wanted Cynthia to gain more value with meaningful results and develop new long-term habits. We proceeded with the visualisations.

With all the noise and buzz going on around us at the gym, Cynthia appeared to be fully on board with the visualisation and her eyes were closed. Naturally, I wasn't privy to know what she was visualising as I gently prodded her with questions about how she was feeling ...

After the visualisation, Cynthia sat there numbly looking like she was going to fall apart. She rushed away from the gym. I wondered if I'd made a terrible mistake and thought that I might not see her again. Perhaps I should have offered her the quick-fix blood pumping option first off!

Cynthia phoned me a few days later and told me that she went to the carpark and had cried. She had been in denial; the visualisations had brought everything to the surface and triggered painful emotions. She had felt shame, guilt and a grieving anger for her perception of lost time.

*On a positive note, she did not want to spend **another** year of waiting for the circumstances to be perfect before making a serious commitment to change. The visualisations helped her face the reality that she needed to take immediate action.*

Once you have done the visualisations, I hope you feel committed to the process of change, starting right now. There is just one more thing to do before we start turning things around.

3. LET GO

Say goodbye to self-criticism and hello to self-love

From this moment, release any self-criticism, negative feelings, blame, shame or excuses. They belong in the past and won't serve you now. It is time to look forward and get moving with an attitude of self-love. If you don't discard those feelings of dwelling on the past, they will stop you moving forward. So, let it go.

Mentally gather up any negative thoughts about yourself as if they were pieces of paper. Screw them up into a tight ball, open the window and throw the ball far, far away. I discussed this with Cynthia as I reflected on what I had to do all those years ago too.

I gave myself permission to ditch the guilt and to hang up my beat-ups and excuses of why I hadn't taken action to help myself with stories like, 'I'm too busy', 'I'm too tired', 'I'm an older mum', 'I've got no-one to help me'. I would have thrown my ball in the direction of the shops—straight into the beautician's hot waxing pot. SPLAT!

If you are lacking motivation or not sure what you need to do or how, then let that go too. This may evolve as you read further on and introduce more physical activity into your life. There are plenty of resources to help you in this book.

Be proud of allowing yourself to feel vulnerable in getting *up close and personal*. This will now open the door to change and new possibilities to view yourself in a positive light. Choose today as the first day of a fresh start on your wellness journey. Not Monday, unless today IS Monday. Congratulations on getting started!

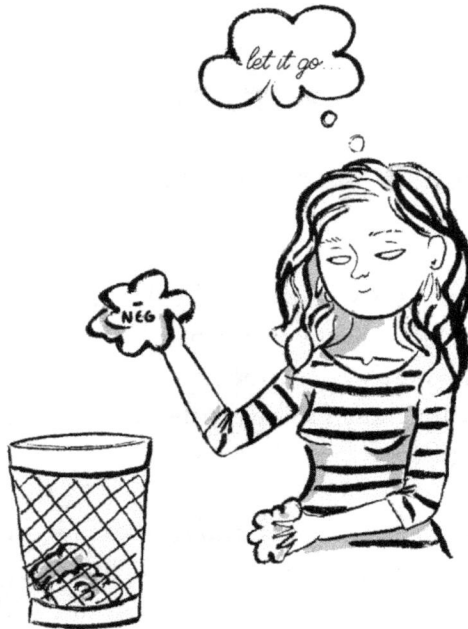

Q&A

Q. What if I feel overwhelmed on all the things I want to change? My list is enormous!

Taking on too much at once can make us feel anxious, wondering how we will ever get it all done. This can cause us to procrastinate and be at risk of inaction. Be reassured, we will start with small steps—it is not necessary to change everything right now!

Q. I just want to lose weight. Do I still need to do the visualisations?

I recommend it as a useful tool to bring more awareness to your emotions and explore perceived failure and success. This generates a greater level of commitment and motivation.

Q. What if I find it hard to let go of my self-criticism?

It is a new skill to practise. You can learn to push back and reframe that internal dialogue to one of self-love and compassion.

IN A NUTSHELL:

- **Look for opportunities** in uncomfortable emotions, which can shed light on your situation.

- **Develop awareness** and identify areas of your health for improvement.

- **Commit to change** by doing the two visualisations and committing to the change process.

- **Let go** and say goodbye to negative feelings and excuses. Mentally bundle them up into a ball and throw away. Choose TODAY as a fresh start on your wellness journey.

CHAPTER 2

Ignite your Inner Spark
Foundations to success

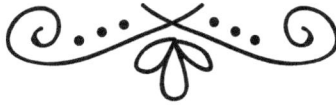

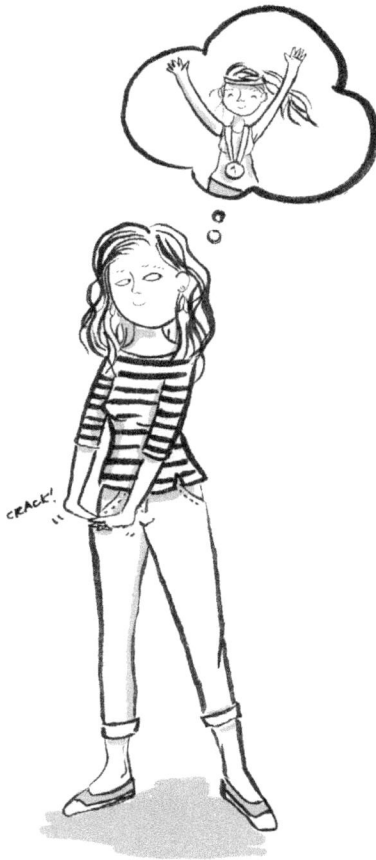

'Begin with the end in mind.'

– Stephen R. Covey

*W*hat do I do now? After developing conscious awareness and committing to the process of change around your health, you may be wondering where to start?

In today's world of fast, instant solutions, it can be tempting to jump straight into a new routine before exploring your WHY reasons in depth, particularly if you are feeling pumped up and ready to roll. You may wonder why this is necessary if you already *think* you know what you want. For example:

*I've joined the gym to get fit because I get puffed out walking to the letterbox, so I already know **why** I want to get fit! Can't we skip the paperwork and 'why' conversation and get on with it? Just point me in the direction of the next available treadmill!*

I have used an example of the gym, but this could relate to any new behaviour change where we finally feel ready to commit to the process and feel impatient to get moving. We want results NOW!

I have observed this scenario at the gym when eager new members join up. They are enthusiastic and proud of finally getting themselves there to take the plunge. There's a little paperwork to get out of the way first. They need to reveal their medical history and medications, *'Have you ever felt light-headed ...?'* Check all the little boxes ... Tick, tick, tick. Almost done. They have a quick chat and set three goals to work on. All organised and sounds good—right? Ready, set ... *'NOW can I get on the treadmill?'* **NO! Hold your horses—not YET!**

I understand their impatience. After all, isn't it important just to get started? Yes, getting started IS fantastic and they can feel proud and confident to take those first steps. There's just one thing ...

Many people will start a new health kick full of enthusiasm and good intent, then quit after a few weeks or months. I have seen these trends at the gym, a few months after the January surge of new sign-ups.

Often those people may keep their membership going long after they quit turning up, at some level believing they will resume, and so statistics can be unreliable.

So why do people quit behaviours linked to a new routine that they had previously thought were a great idea? There are many reasons for quitting, and some of these even happen at a subconscious level. It is beyond my scope of expertise to speculate on the science behind it, however I do have firsthand experience in helping my clients achieve lasting benefits and not quit!

I want to share one of the big reasons that people quit or lose momentum ... *drum roll please!* It is because they have not set up **strong foundations** at the beginning of their journey to bring purpose and meaning to their behaviours and goals. This can be the difference between a quick fix and long-term success.

Okay, so can we quickly set up the 'strong foundations' and get cracking? What ARE they and how much time will it take?

Strong foundations are a framework to set you up for the future, to maximise your success. It involves:

- exploring your own big WHY reason
- creating a VISION
- reinforcing it to your brain
- developing a system which includes goal setting and behaviour change through habits and daily actionable steps.

If you use an effective method of exploring your vision *before* setting goals and practising new behaviours, you are less likely to quit!

This chapter will discuss the importance of investing time to set up your framework to bring more meaning to *why* you want to bring about change. The why questions will not focus on beat-ups and negative emotions of fixing what is wrong, nor do I want them to provoke a quick auto response. Rather, I'm talking about 'why' in the context of positive advantages to change.

Can the real reason please step forward?

Have you ever felt stumped when asked why you want to change some habits around your health and fitness? Sometimes we feel put on the spot and come up with a reason that we think the person asking is expecting. We might also rattle off the first instant answer that comes to us. It may be logical and sensible, but is your reason meaningful or exciting enough to fuel your choices if you lose motivation?

My client, Suzi, came to the gym for personal training sessions. Her general body language was a giveaway as to the discomfort she was feeling and she expressed thoughts of disliking her body. She hid behind a hunched posture and long dark hair. There was no eye contact. Why did she put herself through such anguish when she looked like she didn't want to even be there?

After we chatted, we found a passion of Suzi's—music. She found her voice and told me her desire to gain confidence and her speaking voice.

Suzi became more alive as she spoke from the heart with pure emotion. She was a rock musician in a well-known band. She told me how she had a negative self-image and battled to hide low confidence on stage. She loved singing but hated speaking to announce songs or sets and said the minimum amount of words to get by. She was also shy and battled to converse with strangers.

Suzi was to perform at a major gig and dreamed that this could be her big break.

She had tried to exercise by herself at home, but the isolation was part of her problem. Having this desire to perform well was her motivating force.

I continued to work with Suzi, to expand and dig even deeper with her *why* reasons before helping her to set up a method of reinforcement, which I will share with you in this chapter.

Find your why passion

We don't all have reasons like Suzi! Don't be swayed by someone else's vision or compare yourself with others. Finding your own reasons can be tricky—it means being vulnerable and giving up excuses. Your own reasons are unique and personal. If you can trade *practical* for *passion*, then it's easier to link that heartfelt emotion as to why you want to do something. Your vision will inspire you if it is true to who you are, rather than the who you *think* you should be.

Whether you are embarking on a new health kick like quitting sugar, introducing meditation or starting a fitness program, you will be more likely to succeed in the long term, if you invest a little more of your time and imagination to explore the benefits. This is achieved by creating a **personal wellness vision.**

But didn't we already do this in the visualisation? We *did* look ahead and imagine your future, but this was just a glimpse to get the ball rolling and gain your commitment to start. Now we need to zoom in even closer and explore the benefits AND craft this into a written form VISION to ensure you keep going! It's easy to feel pumped up now or even for a few weeks or months with genuine optimism to achieve a short-term goal. What we need are everyday reasons and positive benefits to be continuously reinforced to our brain, to ensure our new behaviours stick around and become long-term habits.

The wellness vision will shine a light on the pathway forward to help you establish new healthy behaviours, which will develop as habits that you no longer have to even think about. They will become part of your new routine, just like putting on your seatbelt. How good would it feel to have a new fitness or healthy eating routine or daily meditation practice become similarly effortless, just like the seatbelt or famous tooth brushing analogy? This is definitely worth the investment!

The power of emotions

I'd heard that linking stories with emotions and repetition were strong motivating factors for recall, particularly if they were embarrassing, fearful or joyful. Have you ever noticed how vividly you can recall those most embarrassing moments from the past? With 'joyful' in mind, I wondered if this theory could work not just for past memories, but for recalling and reinforcing our future visions with ease. I set out to learn more about the link between our emotions and behaviour and gained valuable understanding from a behavioural change seminar for health professionals, presented by Dr Cam McDonald. Dr Cam is a highly regarded dietitian, exercise physiologist, PhD scholar and leader in health within Australia.

I recall him saying, *'What is the day that you want to wake up and do behaviours that make you less healthy by the end of the day?'* It made me think of the visualisations. This struck a chord and highlighted that when we *choose* unhealthy behaviours, such as zero exercise and junky food, we are actually choosing the very outcome that we *don't* want: Visualisation 1!

Linking the outcome to positive emotions

To choose the best outcome (Visualisation 2), we must associate what we want (good health and wellness) with positive emotions. Why? If we associate exercise or healthy eating with negative emotions, such as, *'I **HAVE** to exercise and live on celery sticks because I don't like my body'*, then every time you get your trainers on for exercise, or pick away at rabbit food, you are subconsciously reinforcing that negative self-image, believing that's why you have to do all those things.

Those beat-up ways of thinking can also contribute to us focusing too heavily on the end goal of fixing something, regardless of how we get there, even if this means depriving or punishing our bodies to achieve it. If we don't value the process of our ongoing wellness journey with positive association, it can become a drag to stay motivated when we feel like we 'have to' and so we don't achieve the expected results. We become more likely to quit, and this can chip away at our confidence and self-esteem.

It is far better to choose your behaviour for positive reasons aligned with your wellness vision, so that every time you exercise or eat celery sticks, you associate that with feeling lighter, vibrant, stronger, calmer, joyful or more energised (whatever your reasons in the wellness vision). When you take small daily baby steps of exercise or good nutrition, even in miniscule amounts, you have the opportunity to celebrate those small wins and grow confidence and feel-good emotions every day, not just at the end of achieving a big goal. These compounding baby steps all add up to achieving the results you desire with confidence and a positive association with your health.

More about your wellness vision

Your wellness vision will contain imaginative stories about your future, to generate excitement and feel-good emotions. It will be reinforced to your mind daily, providing meaning and focus. This helps you persevere when times get tough and will maximise your chance for lasting success, as it brings meaning to your goals and new behaviours. As I wanted it to **spark** an emotive response, I call this the **spark vision method.**

Here are the benefits of your wellness vision, spark style:

- **You get to authentically explore your why**, delving deeper than the first obvious answer, to connect with your heart as well as your head.
- **It will generate super excitement** and high enthusiasm for your wellness journey.
- **It will give you clarity and inspiration to focus** on what matters. This makes it easier to know where to start with setting goals and/or cultivating habits. The vision will become your guiding light to show you what's possible.
- **It will reinforce positivity to your brain by visual reminders**. Your brain likes to protect you from harm and discomfort. By having evidence such as daily visual reminders, we can convince your brain that this is a good idea and reinforce positive change. It will also restore that passion.

What about goals?

A *vision* is different to a *goal*. A vision is a clear image of your desired future and is more open-ended. It is aligned with your personal values and principles and provides purpose and meaning to your why reasons. Goals are the vehicle to make things happen. Goals are set as specific targets that will move you towards your vision. Unlike your vision, which may change focus or expand along the way, goals end at some point. That is why you need to do the vision *first,* to bring meaning to your goals and develop a series of actions, which are perfectly aligned with the vision. Take a look at what Suzi wanted to achieve:

*Suzi wanted to lose 5kg, correct her hunched posture, increase her energy, clean up her diet, improve her skin and be able to have good social skills and confidence talking to people. She also wanted to increase her fitness and know how to use the gym equipment so she could attend the gym on her own. These were great **goals but are NOT her vision!***

Instead of jumping straight into goal setting and exercising, we used the spark vision method. This would generate even more feel-good emotions to keep Suzi's motivation high, particularly if she faced any self-doubt or a setback.

We had to create some stories, even if this meant exaggerating a little by making everything not just exciting, but *very* exciting. Not just fun but *extreme* fun. This method generates positive feelings to spark an emotional response and remind us why we want it so much.

We don't always wake up motivated and our reasons can lose some lacklustre on those days. Setbacks can challenge us or make us quit. We can go for the comfortable route *'Oh it wasn't that great an opportunity after all—maybe next year, the timing will be better ...'*

Suzi's toolbox of strategies included her personal wellness vision, to maximise her chance for success. I asked her a series of questions all designed to uncover the benefits she would have from introducing some new behaviours. I didn't just mean the benefits of success on stage, I meant emotions and stories of how this could play out in her everyday life. I wanted Suzi to enjoy the journey *every day*, whether she achieved her end goal of the performance opportunity or not. Here's a sneak peek of an extract from Suzi's vision:

'I feel supercharged with enthusiasm and confidence on and off stage. I love performing to a packed audience, powerfully belting out tunes that I've written from my authentic self. My energy levels are through the roof and I love how strong and vibrant I feel. I come to the gym on my own and it feels great to help others who struggle like I used to. I feel light, sexy and strong! Rock Star Suzi!'

Now it's your turn

I've broken the spark vision method down into five simple steps, based on coaching techniques that I use with clients.

If you are thinking right now, that you would rather run straight to the treadmill and skip all this vision planning stuff, think again! Ask yourself, are you only after a quick fix …?

Important! Give it a go and **do not skip** this step! It is the big, meaningful reasons that will give you staying power, ongoing motivation and generate excitement about a new possibility!

Here's an overview of what we'll do:
1. Plan for it
2. Create your vision with brainstorming
3. Expand on the benefits of wellness into super fun stories
4. Create your final wellness vision, condensed sentence and trigger words
5. Declare it.

Step 1: Plan for it

Marketing date
It's time to set up that marketing session to sell some cool benefits to your brain. If you don't block off some time in advance and plan it in your diary, it may get pushed aside in the daily humdrum. Set up your environment in a way that allows your mind to be calm, clear and receptive to connect with your heart and imagination. This might be out amongst nature or curled up at home with mood music and essential oils—wherever you feel relaxed and able to focus. Use a pen and paper or notebook to write down your thoughts.

Vision does not always come to us easily—and to do this with the most value, means getting in touch with what's below the surface. Relax your mind and aim to suspend your internal critic. It is not about desiring perfection. It is about envisioning the changes that are important to you in keeping with your unique personal values.

Step 2: Create your future vision

The vision exercises below will help you paint a mental picture of your future life in regard to your wellness. This could be 12 months or longer, and it can be amended at any time.

Brainstorm

Imagine yourself back in Visualisation 2. Zero in on it with more detail and write down how you saw your desired future if you made those changes to your health. What are you doing and what emotions do you feel? What benefits have you experienced?

Brainstorm! Write down words, bullet points, whatever comes to mind. **Just write!**

Instead of saying *'I've lost weight and look good'*, you might say *'I feel light and bursting with energy. I've got my confidence back and am {running} again.'*

Another option is to revisit your **up close and personal exercise** from Chapter 1 and write the **opposite** of those words that described your symptoms or feelings you wanted to change.

For example:

- *'I feel tired, unfit and lacking in motivation'* becomes *'I feel energetic, fit and motivated'*.
- *'I feel heavy and stressed'* becomes *'I feel light and calm.'*

Writing tips

If you have any 'writer's block', then set a timer for five minutes and start writing about another topic which you feel passionately about. Or, try fantasising about your dream holiday, and who you would take if you won lotto! It is like doing a warm-up exercise and can stimulate those creative juices to flow.

If you found this exercise a little formal or stilted, don't worry. This next step will create some fun stories as we explore the benefits. Cynthia found the first exercise difficult due to her confidence about getting the wording right. We persisted and used the simple technique of writing down her opposite words, *'energetic, strong, light, fit, happy, sexy, even-tempered, love myself, proud and confident'*. She then wrote *'I'm happy that I've cleaned up my diet and am exercising regularly, enjoying the challenge. I feel proud that I have taken back control to reclaim my health and happiness.'* This was an okay start, but it needed *much* more oomph to sell it to her brain.

Step 3: Make it more sparky!

The more clearly you can connect with the images and feelings in your vision, the more likely you are to take positive actions towards manifesting it into reality.

'Oomph'

You can now go crazy and add in the oomph or spark factor and build on the positive feelings you wrote about in Step 2.

What are the **advantages** that you will be experiencing from improved wellness? How would those benefits show up in your everyday life? What would you be doing differently that you are not doing now?

To sell this vision to your brain, it needs to look enticing, but within the realms of possibility. Use emotive stories, imagination and creativity. There will be another draft before editing it down in size, so be generous with the amount you write. Go crazy with all the benefits you can think of!

Your reasons will all be unique and different. Once Cynthia started, it was like her pen could hardly keep up with her mind. She took on the oomph factor with great gusto. She wrote pages of real everyday benefits that included what her relationships with her partner and friends would look like, and about reclaiming her passion for teaching. Here is an extract:

'I'm proud of reclaiming my health and feel light, free and energised with more zest for life! I've rediscovered my passion for teaching with a newfound joy. I stand strong and confident in front of my students and they have trust in me like I do in myself. We have fun and laughter in the classroom adding to its positive vibe. I am smiling and feel warm and content and glad in my heart that I didn't give up teaching when I was feeling so unhappy. I choose to be a teacher, the best I can be. I want to savour and enjoy every moment of these last two years of teaching before I retire and explore my new passion for travel and art. I now love shopping for sexy clothes (much to my husband's joy!). Signed, the Passionate Professor.'

To demonstrate how different our visions will be, here are some other extracts:

'I desire to reclaim my confidence at the gym. I want to get out of the corner and feel comfortable. I will feel relaxed with a sense of freedom as I walk around trying out new machines, smiling and greeting other members. I love my new social life and feel a sense of belonging.'

'I see my body responding to my great new healthy eating habits. I blitzed my weight loss goal and dropped ten kilos. In summer I will be proud to step in and out of the swimming pool in a slinky costume without hiding under a baggy t-shirt. I'll definitely be feeling sexy, toned, healthy and proud of myself.'

'I have reclaimed my spiritual practice by meditating every day. I feel calm with more joy and lightness in my life. I am living in the now and have a deeper connection in all my relationships.'

'I was tired of making excuses about starting again on Monday. Now I am proud of prioritising my health and pushing through barriers to make exercise a priority. It's become easy and I love how much energy I have and how it helps me to deal with the demands of a busy life.'

'I have more energy to run around and play games with the kids at the park. I join them in the playground and am trying to master the monkey bars too! I intend to live to an old age and be a healthy grandparent. I want to be a great role model for my children and for them to remember that they had an energetic, cool mum that loved to play with them and had a positive self-image.'

'I nourish my body with beautiful fresh, colourful food and enjoy cooking and sharing it with family and friends. I practise self-control and discipline but also feel okay about having treats. I'm no longer worried about having heart problems and feel good about my body. When I open the wardrobe, I can pick anything out and know that it will fit perfectly.'

Step 4: Final wellness vision

Edit

Revise your list and remove any lukewarm reasons. Every reason, story or feeling needs to be meaningful and earn its place on your final vision. It may sound ridiculous to someone else but mean everything to you within your values. Make your language punchy and sparky. You will look at this often so ensure it inspires you!

After editing:

- Rewrite or type your final (for now) wellness vision. I suggest less than half a page of sentences or bullet points.

- Below that, add a short, condensed version of one or two sentences starting with *'I desire to ...'*.
- Choose a couple of triggers words that will remind you of your vision.
- Make it visually appealing. Some people jazz theirs up with images or a dash of colour. For an electronic version, try an app such as Canva. If you already use a vision board, you could add it to that.

This is an example of Cynthia's shortened condensed version and trigger words:

*'I desire to reclaim my zest for life with passion. I feel light, energetic, fit, focused, joyful, free and proud'. Trigger words: '**Joyful and Free'.***

Step 5. Declare it!

Pin it up
Pin up your wellness vision in a prominent place where you will see it often. Review it regularly to maintain focus on your intentions, to remind yourself why you choose the behaviours that will make it a reality.

Visualise the feel-good reasons why you are on this journey and see yourself in the picture with your vision actualised. Your vision can direct your thoughts, so keep reviewing it until it becomes a part of you. Instead of just reading the words, try and connect with it emotionally.

Reinforce with a trigger
Triggers can link your memory back to the vision. Your trigger could be one or more words, a mantra, a song or a rap. It could also be a visual reminder near your computer, a coloured wristband or a symbol you wear.

Suzi used lyrics from a song to link to her vision. If she needed to bring back the spark, she would play the song or sing a phrase, belting it out loud or silently in her head. She imagined herself as a *Rockstar* with trigger words **'Authentic and Strong'.**

Cynthia imagined herself as the *Passionate Professor* who wanted to reclaim her zest for life. She created her own symbol and logo of the word **ZEST**. She kept her trigger words of **'Joyful and Free'** pinned up by her computer.

Whenever the Passionate Professor finds opportunities to exercise, she inwardly celebrates and reminds herself, *'With every rep and every step, I feel more **Joyful and Free'.*** The trigger words remind her of the feel-good emotions generated from her vision, in turn reinforcing her actions and urging her on.

Share it

Sharing your desires will strengthen your commitment. This could be with a friend, partner, coach or even others who are on the same path.

Q&A

Q. I don't know about my why and find it hard to come up with reasons that excite me.

Ask yourself whether you have any fears or resistance about doing this exercise? If you don't feel confident of being that person in your vision, ask what it would take to build that confidence? You may benefit from help around this from a coach. You could also revisit the exercise on another day.

Q. Do I have to share my why?

No. The initial brainstorming might allow you to be more open if you know that only you will see it, but it can be beneficial to share the final list with people on the same path as you.

Q. What if my vision changes?

It is common for your focus to change as you start to bring in changes. Sometimes what we thought was important can suddenly lose priority. That is why it is important to read your vision regularly and adjust it in line with any change in circumstances or values.

IN A NUTSHELL:

- **Set aside some time** to plan your vision.

- **Do the brainstorming exercise** to create your future vision. Use positive words and emotions.

- **Add in the 'oomph'** factor of super fun stories of the advantages of improving your health.

- **Revise and edit** to create your final wellness vision. Also, add a condensed sentence starting with 'I desire to ...' and a couple of trigger words. Make it visually appealing.

- **Declare it**—pin it up, consider sharing it and set up reminders and triggers.

Right ... after all that brainwork and visualising, it's time to get moving! This next chapter will help you get started!

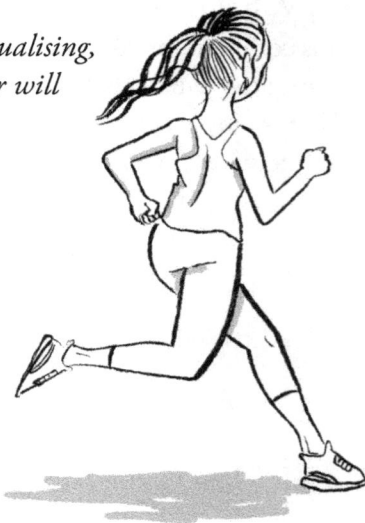

CHAPTER 3

Let's get Physical, Fizzikal! ♪

Getting started with exercise

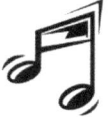

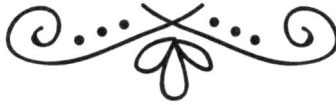

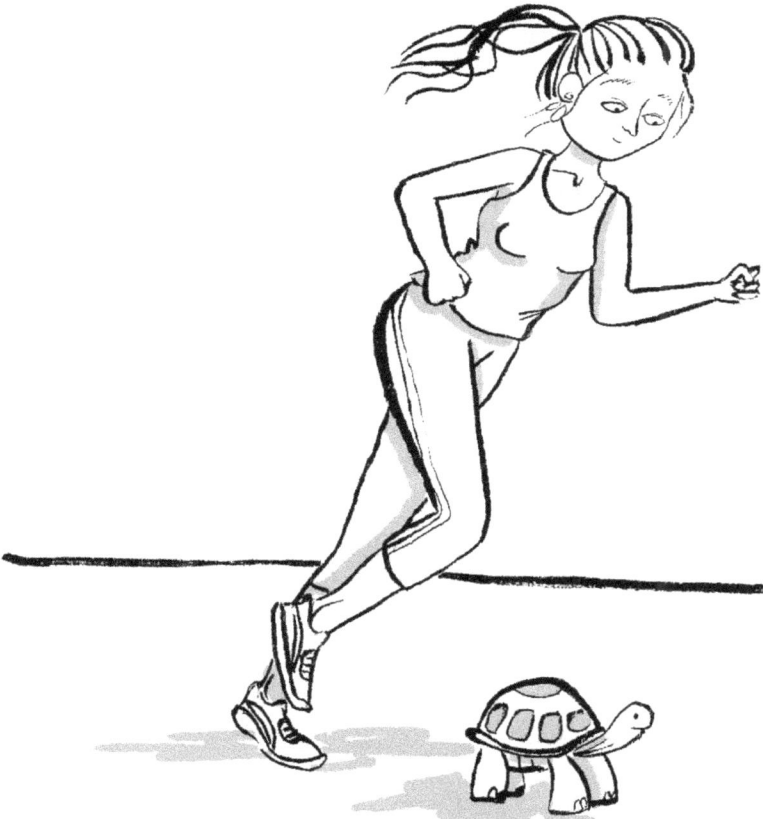

'You don't have to go fast; you JUST have to GO!'
– T. Harv Eker

How do YOU relate to exercise? *'I hate exercise', 'I'm not cut out for it' 'No pain, no gain'...* I've heard it all, and perhaps you have too!

No matter what you believe, being more physically active with exercise can tick off many boxes to achieving optimal wellness. Having started on your foundational framework with your vision now lighting up the pathway forward, let's get cracking and find new ways to enjoy it. We can start moving right now! No more delays, I promise ...

The word *exercise* can generate all sorts of mixed emotions. While some people absolutely love exercise, others hate the thought of all that 'hard work'. I'm here to reassure you that exercise is as simple as you want it to be. It is about increasing your physical activity. It's about movement in a way that causes you to breathe more deeply and cause your heart rate to speed up.

Increasing your physical activity will have wonderful benefits for your health—emotionally, physically and mentally.

Exercise does not mean having to step foot in a gym or break out in a sweat. It is not about *having* to do anything. It is about *choosing* to get more active with:

- **Unstructured exercise (incidental activity).** It is easy to incorporate into your life in small increments that can be undertaken daily. You won't even have to leave home to do it. Example: washing the car by hand, a one-minute sprint to the bus or a quick dash to beat the rubbish truck coming down the street!

- **A planned approach**. There are lots of options for dedicating a chunk of time for planned exercise. For example, going to a gym or a class or taking an early morning brisk walk for the purpose of exercise.

In the *Perfect Health Meditation* podcast, I recall hearing Deepak Chopra talk about restoring balance and wellbeing. He said: *'Conventional wisdom tells us that if we want to find this balance and be healthy, we must take care of ourselves. However, the real secret to long life health is actually the* **opposite**—*we must allow our bodies to take care of us.'*

If you don't have sufficient physical activity in your life, then you are not allowing your body to take care of you. You may also be missing out on experiencing those mood-boosting endorphins that you can feel from exercise. The human body is incredible, and exercise with increased blood flow nourishes the trillions of cells within, allowing them to carry out the jobs they are designed to do.

I want to promote exercise in a positive way but also remind you, that being inactive is a risk factor for developing chronic illnesses such as cardiovascular disease, type 2 diabetes, osteoporosis and some cancers.

The Heart Foundation of Australia reports that:

Coronary heart disease is the leading cause of death in Australia. It claims more lives than any other disease, causing one in 10 deaths.

Regular exercise (and a healthy diet) is one of the best things you can do for your heart health—even as little as 10 minutes of physical activity a day is beneficial.

But that's not all! Exercise is also incredible for mental health, and we know firsthand how happy and energised we feel after a workout. If you really want to get inspired to jump up right now and lace up your running shoes, tune into John J. Ratey, MD, an Associate Clinical Professor of Psychiatry at Harvard Medical School and an expert in neuropsychiatry and the brain-fitness connection. His motivational books and TED talks will really get you moving! In his studies, he has found that exercise is as effective as certain medications in treating anxiety and depression, and as he describes below, it also reduces stress:

'At every level, from the microcellular to the psychological, exercise not only wards off the ill effects of chronic stress; it can also reverse them. Studies show that if researchers exercise rats that have been chronically stressed, that activity makes the hippocampus grow back to its pre-shrivelled state. The mechanisms by which exercise changes how we think and feel are so much more effective than donuts, medicines and wine. When you say you feel less stressed out after you go for a swim, or even a fast walk, you are.'

The social benefits of exercise can be just as significant as the physical activity itself. We can choose how social we want our exercise to be— there's no right or wrong, purely a preference:

- Groups give you accountability, support and more social opportunity to meet others with a common interest. They reduce feelings of loneliness and for many people, the social benefits are the most important.

- Working out on your own can give you a time for solitude and peace and quiet. If you are constantly interacting with people all day long, then it can be a welcome relief to switch off from others.

- You can also have the best of both worlds, by exercising on your own wearing headphones, whilst surrounded by other people. Even just being amongst others in a gym can boost your spirits with a sense of belonging.

Regardless of your current level of fitness, start small with baby steps to build confidence around the changes that you can begin today. Keep reminding yourself of how increasing your physical activity can take you closer to your vision. Let's explore getting started.

1. STARTING POINT – GETTING THE ALL CLEAR

No ifs and buts!

First things first. Is there anything stopping you from building more exercise into your life? If so, NOW is the time to get this sorted!

If you have an injury, disability or health issue, investigate your options. Remember, exercise does not have to mean going to a class or a gym. It needs to be tailored to your own situation and any movement is better than none.

Check in with yourself that you are not using excuses for not being more active. Sometimes our reasons for not starting have nothing to do with the blurb that we rattle off … *'But I don't have time', 'I've got no money', 'I've got a sore shoulder', 'I don't like exercise' 'If only I had someone to walk with'*. Grasp hold of this opportunity to do what you can right now and nourish your body to take care of you. Take the 'ifs and buts' out of your vocabulary and manage what you can.

Your priorities in life will win!

If your issue is not physical, but is time or money, then remember that the priorities that YOU choose, will win. Instead of asking how to fit exercise into your schedule, ask yourself how you can elevate exercise to be a top priority? Today. Not next year when you'll have more time. Same goes for reservations around what you spend money on.

Health assessment

Get an assessment from a health professional if required. This could be to address a physical injury, medical condition or mindset issue. Visiting my doctor before commencing an exercise program not only reassured me that I was safe to proceed, it also helped me to feel committed and accountable.

My visit to the GP

I recall making a long appointment with the doctor before starting formal exercise. It gave me a few days grace to get my head around my fear of burpees! Maybe she could give me a letter excusing me from doing them, like a parent/school note? She popped me on the scales. I'm sure that all doctor's scales are calibrated at 2kg heavier. Doc agreed that a minimum of 10kg would be a good start and 15kg even better. She organised blood and hormone testing, blood pressure and discussed the pelvic floor (a referral to a specialised women's health physio was helpful). I came home with a bundle of brochures and a few of Doc's own tips thrown in. She didn't give me a note but said 'NO to burpees just yet!' Phew—I now had the 'all clear' and was ready for full steam ahead.

Even if you don't have a health problem, it's a timely opportunity to have that regular medical check-up that we are often guilty of putting off. Some of the tests you may want to discuss with your doctor include:

- skin checks
- blood pressure, cholesterol and blood glucose testing
- cervical screening test for women (replaces the pap smear test)
- hormone testing—for women experiencing menopausal symptoms
- bowel cancer screening—free kits are available for eligible Australians between 50 and 74 years of age
- breast cancer screening—two-yearly mammograms are free through BreastScreen Australia for eligible women over the age of 40
- bone density testing—advancing age can increase the risk of osteoporosis, making you more vulnerable to fractures. You might also be tested for vitamin D levels
- pelvic floor education—for further information or instruction on pelvic floor exercises, discuss it with your doctor. A specialised physiotherapist may also help. For men reading this book, yes, you do also have a pelvic floor!

40

The above list is not comprehensive—it can be used as a reminder to talk to your doctor about testing recommended for you, based on your own personal health and risk factors. In addition to the above, if you have been experiencing mood swings or feeling down and irritable, you can also discuss those feelings (and any other mental health concerns) with your doctor too.

2. MAKE A START

Do what you CAN!
While you are busy planning the best exercise for you, get started anyway, in some form. It could be as simple as stretching, walking around the neighbourhood (or the clothesline), running for the bus, swimming, gardening, any type of action that gets you moving.

If you have been very inactive, your aerobic fitness can be poor. Don't despair—try taking more breaks or reduce the pace. If you are concerned about breathlessness or any other issues such as feeling unwell or dizzy, rest up and seek medical advice. You need to pace yourself and build up gradually.

Ask for help!
If you are new to exercise, it can feel uncomfortable to venture into unknown territory, and it can really help to have a buddy or relevant professional to support you. I know this from firsthand experience. I made the mistake of not reaching out for help, thinking I didn't need it and could manage on my own. Once I did say yes to professional help, that short-term boost was all I needed to then go on and take the reins back for myself. To demonstrate, here is the story of how I got back into exercise after the 'grandmother' moment and getting the 'all clear' from the Doc.

I started researching exercise classes like aqua aerobics but loathed the thought of shopping for bathers! I felt a general lack of confidence about joining a fitness class on my own and didn't know anyone at my 'beginner' level to join me.

I wasn't ready to give up and kept thinking of the mirror audit and the alternative if I didn't keep pursuing this. I wondered if I needed to be partially fit to 'qualify' joining an established group? It was becoming even more exhausting just thinking about it and I wasn't sure what to do next. My next thought was to buy some equipment to exercise in the comfort of my own home. I bought a treadmill which eventually doubled up as a clothing rack and dust collector. I also vowed to try out the unopened Pilates DVDs which I had bought on the shopping channel during a 3 am breastfeeding session many months prior.

*With the tiredness I felt, it was becoming all too hard. I had always been so self-motivated, and the thought of calling in professional help seemed unwarranted. **I** was the person who had managed a law firm and a 5-star resort! I'd proved how capable I was—surely, I should be able to do this on my own!*

My husband and well-meaning friends were supportive in the way they thought best. But by telling me that I looked fine and to accept that it was early days after having kids as an older mum, didn't help me feel any better. Physically, I probably did LOOK fine, but inside, I was unhappy and desperately wanting to feel energised. As the weeks rolled on and I still battled to get back into exercise other than walking, I decided I was ready for some outside help.

Opportunity came knocking on my door in the form of a neighbour. BINGO! Was this the universe testing me out to see how serious I really was about reclaiming my health and happiness?

The neighbour wanted to know if I'd like to split some costs and share a personal trainer with some others in the street. She also asked whether I watched 'The Biggest Loser' on TV? I immediately got goosebumps whilst conjuring up images of a boot camp sergeant major wearing a military vest and yelling at me to do more burpees! I had no idea how to even DO a burpee and I was excused from them anyway! I was out of options having exhausted my solo attempts. I said YES.

Day one of training: I rummaged through my clothing to find something stretchy and black to hide my muffin top. I was expecting a 6-foot tall, scary, Arnie look-alike with bulging muscles. Instead, I was pleasantly surprised to meet the new trainer, Mel. She came in the form of a stunning, 5-foot-4, fitness model look-alike, with a mop of blonde dreadies. She was young—late 20s, wholesome-looking and the picture of good health. For a fleeting moment, I wondered what she could possibly know about a 45-year-old first-time mum who'd had three hours sleep? Wrong! My mind changed instantly as she smiled. It was dazzling and friendly. Her clear blue eyes conveyed empathy and understanding as she listened mindfully to what I said. I hoped she wasn't psychic and read my mind of first impressions! Mel had me feeling instantly at ease, and I felt that this could be my ticket to freedom. Bring on the burpees baby—I'm in!

Let the fun begin … step-ups. Mel understood that doing a step up to the park bench was totally outside my current capabilities. I did mine on the tiny step in the children's playground, all of eight inches high! I didn't feel like a biggest loser, I felt accepted and was on the path.

I was ecstatic! I had started, and we'd chatted and laughed and exercised. I wanted to skip home with joy, although my pelvic floor wasn't quite up to it yet. I had those incredible endorphins running through my body and when I got home, felt like I'd been away on holiday and it had only been an hour. What fantastic medicine this was. I could hardly wait for our next session to feel this way again. And I did, every week and every month until I spread my wings and ventured out on my own.

I'd started out to lose weight and get my body strong, but the focus was now about feeling great and having that twice-weekly 'holiday'. The energy that was running through my body (even after sleep deprivation) was like waking up out of a dark winter hibernation and discovering spring for the first time.

My body responded well. I made better choices around food because I had more energy to shop and cook, and I wanted to nourish my body to provide fuel for the burpees! The weight came off naturally and I bought new sporty clothing that I felt good in. I had my mojo and my confidence back. I loved the social aspect of exercising with the other ladies too. I also became a happier wife and mum because I was joyful on the inside and proud of overcoming the challenges I'd faced.

With my confidence restored and a thirst for a new challenge, I ventured out to exercise classes and activities on my own. This was incredible. Not only had I turned the corner, I became unstoppable! Surely there were other women out there like I had been, struggling in isolation, and they needed to know that it's okay to ask for help. It was at that time that I obtained my Certificate III & IV in Fitness and become a personal trainer. I chose not to return to the corporate life behind a desk. I felt alive and wonderful and wanted to share it with everyone!

PS. Fifteen years on, my beautiful friend and trainer, now resides in Margaret River (minus her dreadies which she cut off for charity) and is now a fabulous mum in her 40s. Thank you, Mel. You came into my life at the precise time that I was ready for change and receptive for help.

Reflecting back, I wish that I had consulted a physio or fitness specialist much earlier but feel fortunate that a neighbour knocked on my door that day. If you need help, then ask for it. There's no need to do this on your own and the sooner you start, the better.

3. GET PREPARED

What do you need?
Time to ditch the old baggy t-shirt, trackydacks or saggy bathers and smarten up with clothing that helps you to feel good. Women should also invest in a supportive sports bra.

Shoes
Good shoes are a must! The old pair of Dunlops may be great in the garden or for a gentle stretch session (bare feet may even be better) but won't cut it out on the walking track. Supportive shoes are going to help your body with alignment and minimise ankle rolling and possible injury. However, when you start looking, it can be easy to feel overwhelmed at the choice and range of trainers all marketed to us for a single purpose.

If you want to start a walking program, then a walking or running shoe will be a great choice as they are generally light with good spongey shock-absorbing features, designed to absorb the impact of your weight on the ground. If walking turns into a bush hiking adventure, then walking boots will give you more stability on uneven ground. Seek good advice from a dedicated sports shoe retailer and discuss your needs and budget.

Music
Create fun, motivational playlists of music to help pick up the pace in time with the beat. I use the Spotify app and have set up a range of playlist options to match the mood or tempo I want on that day.

Techy stuff
Tracking and training apps, workout timers, sports watches, heart rate monitors, pedometers and Fitbit type activity trackers are optional extras, if you like to incorporate technology to your workout. I often choose music or 'a la naturale' background over tech, but apps like the original 'Couch to 5K' which I've used are good, particularly if you have a specific goal in mind. You can continue to listen to music

45

with the added benefit of a virtual coach that instructs you when to run, walk, jog or stretch. There are many similar apps available that include video demonstrations of exercises, so try out some of the freebies first and ask around for recommendations.

Invest in comfy workout headphones that are secure-fitting and resistant to sweat. A portable speaker is a great option too for use at home or for those garage workouts.

Diary
Choose a traditional or digital version but ensure those planned sessions go in your diary.

Other
Water bottle, towel and dedicated gym bag and any other bits and pieces you need for the activity.

Equipment
Don't get carried away in the shopping sales. I recommend only buy what is necessary at the time. If you are considering some large pieces of equipment, for example a treadmill or bike, it can be a good idea to hire for a couple of months first to ensure it will not end up like mine. For an inexpensive indoor cardio option, try the not so dorky mini trampoline rebounder (reminiscent of the 80s). I love using mine when I need a quick burst of exercise away from the computer. The current models have handles to hold on to.

Requirements for home workouts are minimal, and you can achieve great results by using your body as the resistance or use a homemade option of sand-filled plastic bottles. If you want to buy a few small items, consider an exercise mat, resistance bands, dumbbells, fitball and a skipping rope.

For less than $60, I recommend a **foam roller,** which is a lightweight, cylindrical tube of compressed foam. My 'best friend'—it is *not* a 'torture tool', can be used for self-massage and myofascial release to help relieve muscle tightness. It is an effective postural tool to counteract hunching over a computer or phone—every teenager needs one too! The roller is versatile and can be paired with bands and weights or is perfect to relax on and practise calm breathing techniques before bedtime.

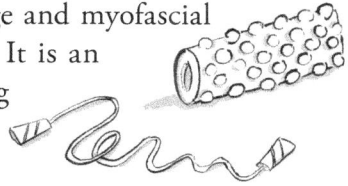

4. FINDING THE PERFECT FIT OF EXERCISE FOR YOU

Exercise is for *everyone* so find the perfect fit for you. It's great if you can have the added benefit of enjoying the activity.

To get as many benefits from exercise as possible, try and incorporate the following four main types of activity, depending on what your body needs most. It's advisable to have this assessed by a fitness or medical professional who can tailor a specific program for you.

Cardiovascular: Cardio activities improve heart and lung health and build endurance to increase your level of fitness. This type of exercise can be 'aerobic' using oxygen to fuel your muscles, for example walking, or 'anaerobic' (without oxygen) such as short sprints. Aim to get your cardio fix every day with moderate intensity activities that increase your heart rate but don't make you breathless, as well as vigorous high intensity activities that require more effort and make you 'huff n puff'. You will fire up your metabolism to keep a healthy weight and experience brain and mood-boosting benefits too.

Strength or resistance training: Perhaps you feel you don't need it? You appear strong enough to carry out daily activities … so why bother? In addition to building and preserving your muscle strength, it is a key factor that works to increase bone density, which helps you to stay strong as you age. Strength training can also increase your metabolism and is just as important for your overall health as doing cardio. Aim for 2–3 sessions per week and use weights and bands or your own body weight as the resistance.

Stretching, flexibility and mobility exercise: Daily stretching is so beneficial for our health and improves our flexibility of muscles and mobility of joints. It also helps with posture, relaxation and recovery. Stretching will assist you to perform other types of exercise, improve your agility and minimise your risk of injuries.

Balance training: Balance training exercise helps to improve stability and body awareness and can prevent injury from the risk of falls. It also challenges your core muscles and gives you bonus laughter and relief from boredom as you master new balancing skills. Incorporate single leg activities and give the 'bosu' a test drive!

TIPS for unstructured exercise

Look for the opportunity to add incidental exercise into everything—from household chores to how you get around. Try and include as many of the four main types of exercise as possible.

Crazy example: hanging out the washing

Pop on your wacky imagination glasses for this one … place the washing basket on the ground instead of the trolley. Build leg **strength** through squats to pick up the items and promote **flexibility** with energetic reaches to peg it. Squats could even be elevated to 'squat jumps' for a touch of **cardio**! Want more? Using your non-dominate hand to peg the washing **(brain training)** will take this exercise to a whole new level.

Be warned, you may even start a new neighbourhood craze once they've seen how much energy you have squat jumping by the fence!

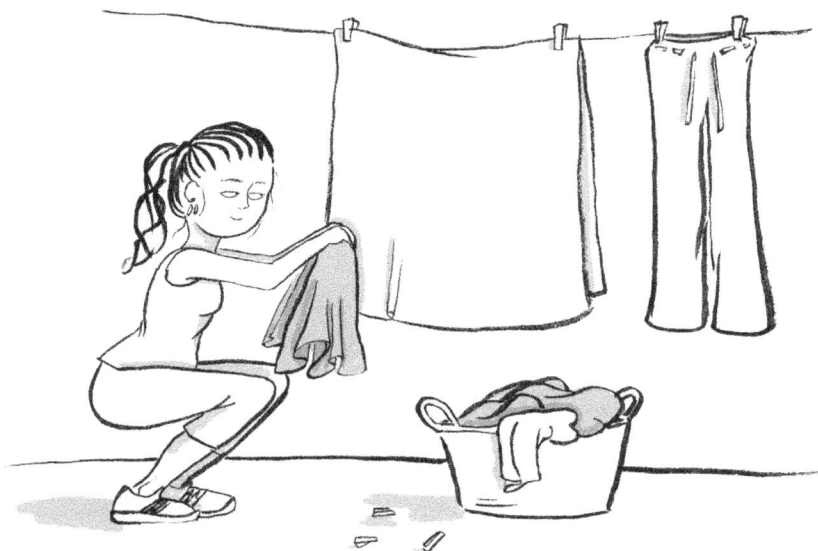

Here are some more ideas:

- practise circus skill balances in the ad breaks
- stretch or rebounding breaks from the computer
- walk or run the dog—*don't have one?* Borrow the neighbours!
- dust n dance, vigorous vacuuming, manic mopping; music cranking!
- brisk walks or sprints to get to the bus even when there's no need to rush
- park your car ridiculously far away from the shops, or better still, ride the bike or walk
- look for ALL opportunities to stand rather than sit, even giving up your seat on the bus for a teen!
- knock out a few squats or push-ups to the kitchen bench when you are waiting for the kettle to boil
- use the stairs whether you need to climb high or not—they will really elevate your fitness and tighten your butt and thighs!

The physical benefits you can get from these activities include improvements in cardio fitness, muscle strength, joint mobility, flexibility, balance and coordination.

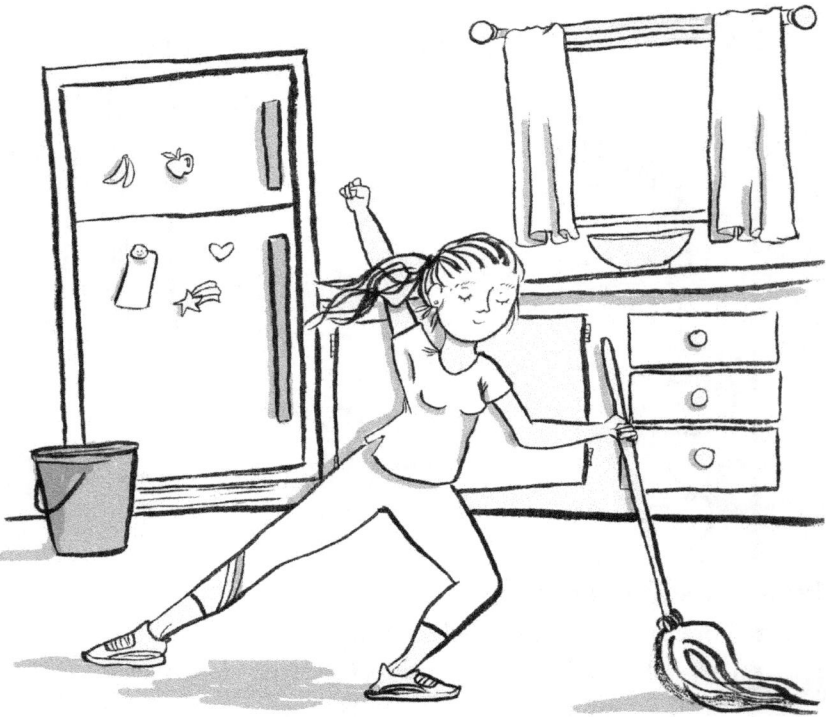

TIPS for planned exercise

With so many options for exercise available, a good first step is to narrow down your choice to the activities you enjoy the most.

Asking yourself the following questions can help you decide where to start:

- What do you need more of—cardio, strength, flexibility or balance? Some activities will incorporate all four components, and others just one.
- Do you prefer a solo workout or exercising in a group setting?
- What timetable will fit into your schedule?
- Do you like a fun factor or are you more results-driven?

- Do you enjoy music within a class?
- Are there any physical, mental or age considerations to factor in? Some classes are tailored for specific areas of the population and different abilities.
- Do you like variety? Some classes offer a fixed routine whilst others are freestyle.
- If you're not doing a home workout, how far would you have to travel?
- Do you have a preference for indoor or outdoor training? Consider sensitivity to weather and environmental conditions.
- Which exercise options will fit into your budget? Remember, walking or swimming in the ocean are free.

Choosing planned exercise

To arm you with more knowledge about the range of choice available, here are some ideas to consider. This list is not exhaustive and is just a taster to help you explore social exercise further.

Gyms: Most gyms are fully inclusive and are for everyone of all ages. Some offer other services such as classes, courses, personal training, swimming and social activities. We'll talk about gyms in more detail in the next chapter.

Studios: Boutique-style studios offer more personalised service and often have a community feel and smaller classes. This allows instructors to give more individualised help by correcting technique. They will most likely know your name too! Try hitting those muscles with a fun freestyle option or rock up to the barre, (yes, the ballet one) and try the popular 'barre' class that is inspired by elements of ballet, Pilates and yoga.

Physiotherapy practices: Many have expanded their services beyond rehab to incorporate education and preventative solutions. A physiotherapist will tailor the workout to suit your abilities, individually or within a small group. It can also be a cost-effective option if the classes are covered under private health insurance—make some enquiries if you think you may qualify.

Personal training: Usually a one on one style of training but it can also include partner and small group training. The sessions will be individually tailored. You can find out more about personal training in the next chapter.

Boxing clubs and martial arts: 'Boxing for fitness' based on traditional boxing is offered by many fitness providers. Don't be shy in trying it out or think it is too 'aggressive'. I've had many clients do a 360-degree change of mind after their first *jab cross hook*.

Group fitness: Choosing can be tricky with so many options available. Group fitness appeals to a wide market—there's catchy music, snappy choreography and it's social and fun. You'll know what I mean if you've ever seen the queues of loyal followers waiting to go into a Les Mills 'pump' or 'spin' class. Try out the many other pre-choreographed and freestyle group fitness classes on offer, including small groups, interval and circuit training.

Aqua classes: Exercising in the water is an ideal low impact workout and is also challenging and fun. Styles vary from high-intensity aqua bootcamp and water aerobics through to relaxing float-fit. Some classes are in shallow water whilst the deep-water sessions use floatation devices. Aquatic dumbbells, noodles and other equipment can add to the level of intensity and enjoyment.

But wait, there's more ...

Dance-style exercise: In 2009, the licensed Latin American Zumba movement took hold and still continues in popularity. There are many other dance-inspired classes which have a fun social element and include throwback hits from other eras. One of my current faves is 'move-fit' with its 'Boogie wonderland' feel and lights off approach. Another on my list to try is 'Clubbercise', which is also taught in a darkened room with disco lights and glow sticks!

Yoga classes: Yoga has stood the test of time in the popularity stakes and has evolved to become even more specialised to cater to various ages and preference of style. Yoga ticks off many boxes incorporating conscious breathing techniques, strength, flexibility and other physical and mental benefits. If you tried it previously and didn't like it, or found it too slow (or fast), try another type of yoga or different instructor. Some fitness centres even offer yoga classes on a surfboard in the pool!

Pilates: Offered in purpose-built studios, physiotherapy practices and fitness centres, there are many variations of Pilates to try. Incorporating flexibility, muscular tone and strength with an emphasis on the 'core' muscles of your body, some classes include small equipment such as resistance bands, whilst other classes use an apparatus called the reformer.

Tai chi and qigong: Don't be fooled by thinking they are lightweight options that don't make you breathless. They might look easy, but you need to try them to appreciate the top physical and mental benefits they offer.

The great outdoors: Australia has an endless offering of beautiful parks and beaches, so outdoor fitness is a popular option. Boot camp is a common sight and was once known as a high-intensity military style of training. Don't be scared of its former 'toughen up' reputation as it has matured into a well-structured option with varying degrees of intensity with no military vests in sight!

Sporting clubs and groups: There are many to choose from and part of the fun is trying new activities in a social setting. In recent years, many sporting clubs have gone through a cultural shift, such as bowling clubs, who have changed their rules to invite everyone onto the green and offer barefoot options too. Tennis does not have to be a formal game, set, match either, with circuit-style cardio classes also on offer.

Online fitness classes: Virtual classes have proved popular during the recent pandemic and saved the day for many who could not leave their home. It is a significant advantage to be able to train from the comfort of your own lounge room, when it suits you.

Fun runs, challenges and charity events: These are social and fun and will encourage you to stay motivated and focused, knowing there is an end point within reach. For example, 21 or 30-day online challenges like push-ups are great because they start small, add on reps every day and you can cheer each other on.

Create your own challenge: Why not organise your own challenge with a group of friends? You could set up a Facebook group and start a mini competition over 14 days. For example, you could commit to doing 30 minutes of different exercise every day and cut out added sugar or alcohol. You could even get your friends to pay an entry fee that could go to the winner or donate to a worthy cause.

The choices are endless. Whether you would like to try tai chi in the park, rowing, bushwalking, paddleboard surfing or wiz around the rollerblade rink, challenge yourself to try a different activity and master a new skill. Start a wish list and enjoy ticking them off. Create your own 30-day challenge to try as many new activities as possible in that time!

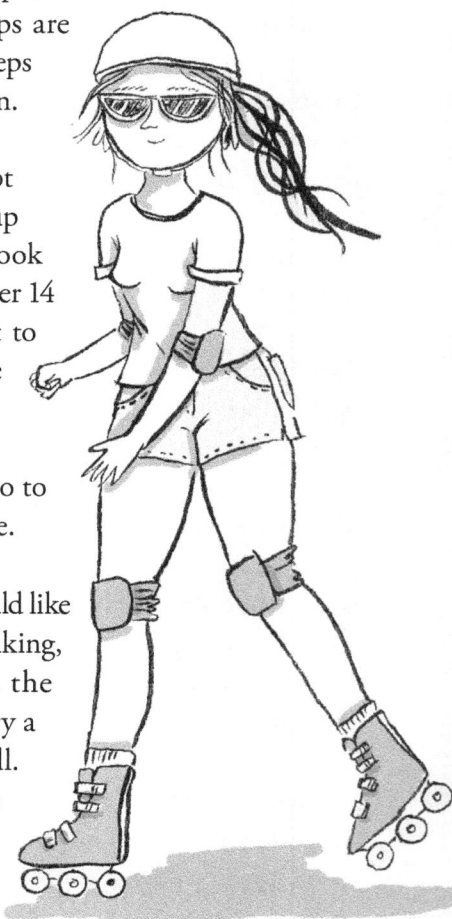

To find out which activities are offered in your local area, you can search online, check community newspapers and noticeboards, contact your local council or visit your closest community centre. You can also ask others for recommendations, in person or via social media, and the Fitness Australia website contains a register of categorised group exercise classes, fitness instructors and personal trainers. Facebook groups can also be a handy place to find a training buddy too.

Q&A

Q. I'm worried that if I join an exercise group, I won't be able to keep up or won't be coordinated.

Start small and gain confidence. Find a class with beginner's options and mention any concerns to the instructor. Listen to your own body and don't do a movement if it doesn't feel right for you. The last thing you need is an injury because you were trying to blend in and do what everyone else was doing, even if it was out of your current range.

Remember, it is not a competition and there are plenty more options. You could also engage a personal trainer to instruct you on some basic moves and correct your posture and breathing. This will help you transition to a group setting. Coordination will improve the more you persist and remember, you won't get better by staying at home.

Q. What if I don't have the time for exercise? I'm so busy!

Be realistic and do what you can. It is also a matter of priorities. Priority will win. Would you manage more exercise if you won $1,000 jackpot each time? Would you do it if you had to pay out $1,000 each time you didn't turn up to exercise? What *would* it take for you to treat exercise as a priority?

Here is the best reason: your life depends on it! Imagine your doctor saying that you could prevent a life-threatening illness from causing your death by committing to a regular exercise program. Would YOU do more exercise if your life depended on it? (Answer) That's a YES!

Q. What if I can't afford to exercise?

There are lots of free options and incidental activities to do. If you want personal training or classes, is there a way to cut back on other things like coffees or manicures? Or can you rejig the budget? Is there a way to share some costs with others? Can YOU be the one to knock on your neighbour's door? Talk to a personal trainer for ideas. Contact fitness training schools. New trainers may offer low-cost options whilst they gain more experience. Depending on your situation, you may be able to set up a reciprocal 'swap skills' arrangement with a trainer.

Q. I don't have anyone to mind my kids and childcare is expensive.

You can involve the kids with your fitness, particularly incidental activity. If you prefer a class, then some fitness providers will encourage you to take children with you because they specialise in that format. It's also an opportunity to share more family time together in a healthy setting. Many clubs have great crèche facilities.

An extra note for mums with young children: I had previously put up barriers about the mornings being too hectic and a husband that travelled. After my husband noticed how happy I was with my new exercise regime, he made it a priority to get home from work as early as possible on those evenings that I exercised. When he travelled, I always found a way to continue. As I valued exercise more than manicures and cappuccinos, I put that money towards babysitting. Occasionally, I would take the kids to training, but I also loved to have more ME time and was a much more patient mum after my sessions. I utilised crèche and kids club programs whilst having a swim, a class or a game of tennis and the costs were affordable.

A final word for women

Women respond to exercise differently than men, particularly in their tolerance and response to hormone fluctuations. Just like the menstrual cycle, the peri-menopausal and menopausal years come with challenges that may include hot flushes, change in body shape, sleep disruption and a change in emotions. An understanding trainer will take this into account and may modify the intensity of the session. When in a class, make your own adaptations and don't feel compelled to keep up with the group.

The pelvic floor can be weakened with age, inactivity or after childbirth. If you feel 'heaviness' or leakage when exercising, then consult your doctor. Be aware that some traditional exercises, including certain versions of sit-ups and crunches, can put more pressure and strain on a weak pelvic floor and can lead to issues such as dysfunction, incontinence and pelvic organ prolapse. Good advice in this area is essential.

On another note, straining from constipation can also add stress to the pelvic organs and nerves. Giulia Enders, in her book *Gut,* gives an amusing and informative look at how to sit on the throne with your feet on a low footrest. The book is a helpful resource on many aspects of our inner workings and written in a humorous and entertaining way.

IN A NUTSHELL:

- **Seek advice from a doctor or health professional** before commencing a new exercise program.

- **Find opportunities for incidental exercise**, to get more movement into everyday activities and reduce the amount of time you are sitting.

- **Research planned exercise** options and diarise. Ask a buddy to join you or consult a fitness professional.

- **Get prepared** for exercise with the right clothing and supportive shoes. Address time management, family routines and anything else you need to do to make exercise happen. Buy a foam roller!

- **Make a start** as soon as you can with baby steps and don't be shy in asking for help.

- **Challenge yourself** to try as many new activities as possible!

CHAPTER 4

Navigating the Gym Jungle and Personal Training
Insider's tips for beginners

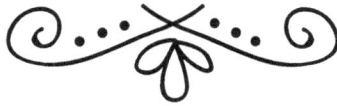

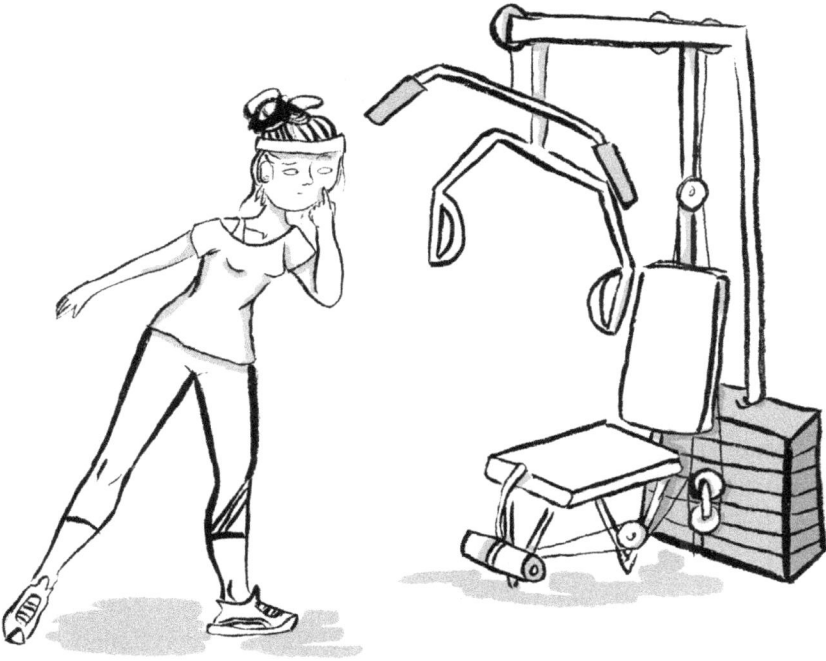

'If you want something you've never had, you must be willing to do something you've never done.'

– Thomas Jefferson

The gym can be a scary place with rows upon rows of machines and contraptions. I used to think so, as I viewed it from the *other* side of the glass windows. Through the lens of my distorted goggles, *everyone* looked fit, pumping it out and moving between equipment with purpose and confidence. My experience with gyms had been limited mostly to classes, the sauna, spa and pool where I could float around in the leisure lane and wonder if I could ever belong in a place like that.

When I did finally decide to take the plunge out of the pool into the gym, I tried to blend in and look confident as I made my way straight to the bike in the corner, wishing I was invisible. I jumped on to find the seat was really low and my knees were practically hitting my chin but I pedalled on anyway, whilst discreetly trying to figure out how to put the seat up without drawing attention to myself. Then there was the tension adjustment to fiddle with ... A few deep breaths and then UH OH! I'd been spotted! A gym instructor was walking the floor and he was heading straight for me ...

I don't know why I felt this was such a problem because after he casually came and said, 'Hi' and helped me find the secret lever to adjust the seat height, I felt a hundred times better and was now best friends with the bike and possibly also with the fit-looking trainer too.

If you lack confidence going into a gym, you are not alone. Here are some of the common reasons that newcomers won't ask for help:

- they are embarrassed about how they look
- they may experience social anxiety when talking to people
- they worry that a pushy salesperson will try and sign them up for a program
- they don't want to appear silly for not knowing what to do, nor do they want to draw attention to themselves
- they feel as if they *should* know how to navigate their way around equipment—after all, everyone else is doing so effortlessly.

If you are worrying about standing out as 'not fitting in' this is precisely the time when you need a little help and encouragement. If you don't ask for help, you might flounder on your own, feeling out of your depth. It may be the first and last time you go to the gym saying, 'Oh I tried it once, but it wasn't for me'.

If you have close access to a gym or personal trainer, find out about them. Visit the gym, ask questions, check out reviews. Look up personal trainer profiles online and ask around your circles for any recommendations or tips. Any extra knowledge will help improve your confidence to take the next step.

Today, gyms are inclusive and open to all ages and abilities, however, this wasn't always the case. Gyms have gone through a huge culture shift since the 1960s and 70s when most were the domain of men who focused on bodybuilding and strength training, rather than exercising for good health. This was often an intimidating environment for women, and it's great to see that gyms have revamped their décor and setup to reflect that cultural shift.

The vibe in gyms can vary from looking (and sounding) like a nightclub through to modern light and bright. It is common to find a combination of heavy-duty industrial equipment alongside pink yoga mats, thus appealing to all. Gyms also vary the look and sound at different times of the day to appeal to various age brackets, so investigate what you prefer.

In addition to the equipment and classes, personal training is available on site within most gyms. It can truly be tailored for everyone and does not need to be confined to the gym environment. There are a variety of options, including home visits and online sessions where you don't even need to leave the house.

In the sections below, I have shared some insider's knowledge to address some of those common concerns about the gym, personal training and group fitness, particularly aimed at beginners.

1. THE GYM JUNGLE

We know that the gym is not for everyone. It may or may not be the best option for you, but if you don't give it go or another try, then you could be missing out on the key that opens up a whole new world that you are yet to discover. If you still have reservations or unanswered questions, here are some tips that may help:

- If you are going to the gym for the first time, take a friend or enquire at reception for a tour. You can call ahead and pre-book or just show up and ask for a look around. You will generally find gym staff very helpful and happy to accommodate newcomers.
- Remember, the gym is not reserved for people of a certain age, sex or body size. Try it out for at least a month or two for a fair assessment. Many gyms will give you a one-week free trial or a low-cost introductory offer.
- Keep in mind that your experience will differ between gyms and also vary depending on the time of day you go. Quite often you will find that mornings can be busy with a cross-section of ages. Lunchtimes are generally quieter, whilst late afternoons and evenings can be busy with students and the after-work crowd.
- If you do a trial run for a week, engage socially with other gym-goers for their unbiased view.
- Always take a towel or two and a water bottle with you. For hygiene reasons, the towel will be used to place on and wipe down equipment. Most gyms supply anti-bacterial wipes, so you can clean any equipment before and after use.
- Every gym has its own unique rules and standards so become familiar with them. Don't feel pressured to sign up for a membership on the day you are shown around. Some gyms have a joining fee and payment plans will vary from the ability to pre-pay up to one year, through to direct debit systems. Ask about cancellation fees and suspension if you are ill or away on holiday.

- If the gym is not for you, feel happy that you have challenged yourself to try something out of your comfort zone and move on to explore your next option. Personal training, anyone?

2. BUDDY UP WITH PERSONAL TRAINING

Throughout this book, I have promoted the many advantages of having a personal trainer. It made such a difference to my training and I only wished that I'd had the courage to book in with one much sooner!

Perfect match

Everyone's experience will be different, and it is imperative that you have the right match of trainer in personality and expertise, for what you require.

It can be nerve-racking turning up for your first PT session. I've had clients confess to me that they had felt like a kid on their first day of school. There can be anxiety around whether a personal trainer is going to push them too far outside their comfort zone or whether they will be capable of doing what they have seen others do. I sometimes meet potential clients in the coffee shop for an informal meet and greet to assess our mutual suitability, and to set their mind at ease.

It's important to feel comfortable with your personal trainer so that you can communicate with them on any worries you have. Most trainers will ask how they can best help you and give you some background info about themselves—this helps to build that rapport. They will discuss your health status, level of fitness, your diet, lifestyle and medications before getting on to preference for exercise and planning the exciting journey ahead.

Personal trainers in Australia require a minimum qualification of a Certificate IV in Fitness. It is also desirable for trainers to have a professional membership with one of the Australian registering bodies, such as Fitness Australia, who oversee the industry and support trainers with ongoing professional learning and access to professional indemnity, public liability and product liability insurances. You may be covered for insurance within a gym facility, but check that an independent personal trainer in their own facility or outdoors also has the appropriate insurances.

A personal trainer will partner up with you to encourage and explore your own potential in achieving goals. Those goals are not exclusive to how fit you want to be and can be for a variety of reasons.

Tips for choosing a personal trainer:
- you can't beat word of mouth—ask for recommendations
- go undercover and watch personal trainers in action. Discreetly, observe how a trainer engages with their clients through body language
- ask if a 'taster' trial session would be possible
- find a trainer that is busy, which is often a good sign
- choose a trainer that specialises in your area of interest such as strength and conditioning, sports specific, rehabilitation, beginner programs, women's health (including pregnancy) and other specialty age groups or considerations.

On top of this, a great personal trainer will have good communication skills, be energetic and motivational, and display empathic listening. They will also be flexible in adapting a session if you are having an off day, or are sleep deprived, and will feel comfortable in referring you on if they are not the best person for the job.

Etiquette
Personal trainers will each have their own guidelines to ensure sessions run smoothly. Some of the common ones include:

- avoid eating a large meal 1–2 hours before exercising
- if you are unwell, call your trainer to discuss alternative plans

- be punctual—most trainers prefer you to get to your session early to do a warm-up first, so check on individual requirements
- take a towel and a water bottle to your session and stay well hydrated by drinking adequate water, prior, during and post training
- if you need to cancel a session, give your trainer as much notice as possible, ideally 24 hours. If you are tired or carrying an injury, contact the trainer in advance so they can adapt the session previously planned
- be consistent and pre-book your sessions in advance. There will be times when you don't feel like it, but if it's prearranged, you are more likely to turn up and feel happy that you did
- tell your trainer about any mindset issues so that they can assist you with this. Communication is a two-way street and the basis for a trusting relationship
- wear comfortable activity clothing, training sports shoes and minimal jewellery. I prefer clients to wear a fitted type singlet when doing a postural analysis. This is also important for weight loss clients when a tape measure might be used
- most importantly, ENJOY your personal training session! All you have to do is turn up with your towel, drink bottle and a willing attitude. Let the trainer do the planning whilst you switch your thinking mind off.

3. FITNESS CLASSES

Group classes are a great way to interact socially and get moving. As mentioned in the previous chapter, the options are endless. From high-intensity workouts like boxing or Zumba, to quieter activities like yoga or tai chi, there is something to suit every age, taste and ability.

The variety and accessibility of classes provide a great opportunity to try something new, under the guidance of an instructor. Challenge yourself to get out of your comfort zone and see where it takes you.

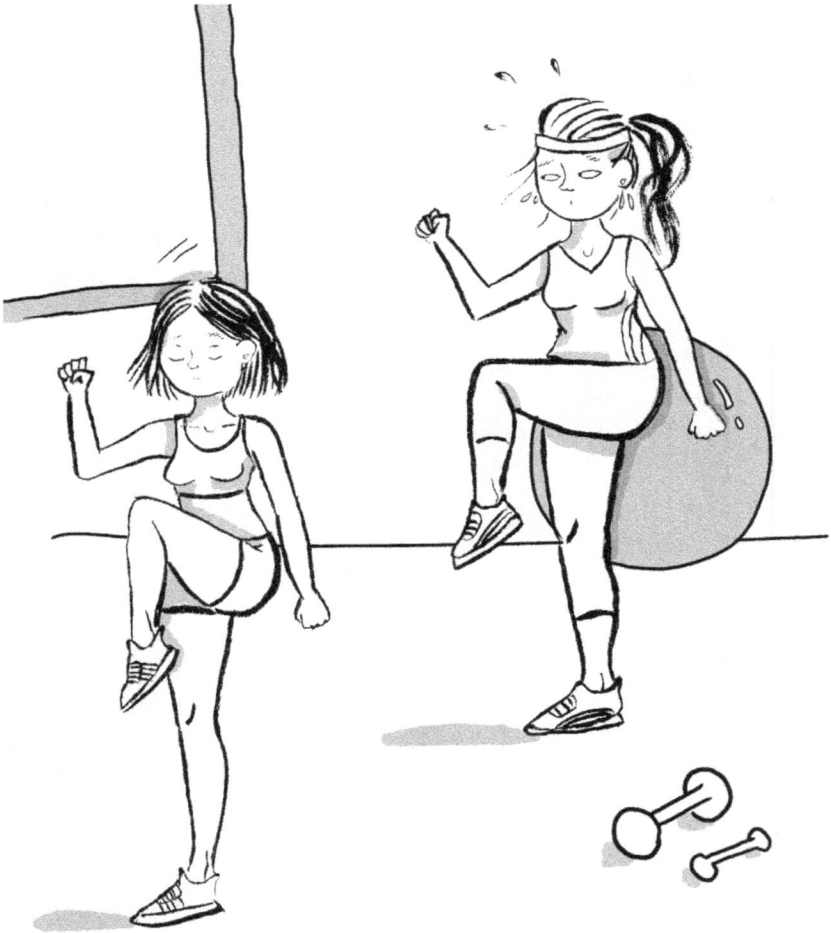

Tips for attending a class in person

Just like the gym and personal training, your first time in a group class can have you feeling a little apprehensive or nervous. Gather information on the class you are attending in the lead-up, so you have an idea of what to expect. The tips below may also provide some reassurance and insight so you can arrive mentally prepared and ready to go.

Do:
- pre-book into the class
- arrive 10 minutes early
- take a towel and a water bottle
- have your phone on silent or do not take it with you
- if it's your first time to a class, let the instructor know
- if you want social engagement, talk to other participants whilst waiting
- advise the instructor of any injuries that they NEED to know about, such as something that might prevent you from participating fully. They can often give you alternative options or adjust the level
- place yourself behind a participant who looks like a regular
- remind yourself that it is not a competition—do only what you can
- congratulate yourself for going to a new class
- look for positives even if you don't like the class or the instructor. Keep trying!

Don't:
- think that people are staring at you
- be put off if others seem fitter or more coordinated than you. They may have been attending that class for years and were also a beginner once too!

Q&A

Q. What if I want to try a class or trainer but there are none close by and I don't have transport?

Enquire whether a mobile instructor can train you at home or consider online classes. You will still get great social and accountability benefits.

Q. Should I engage a female or male trainer?

This is your personal preference. Don't be limited in thinking that a male trainer will not understand women's issues. What counts most with any trainer, is their level of professionalism, knowledge in specialty areas and communication skills.

Q. I've found classes to be boring and yet they are usually booked out. Is it just me?

Fortunately, we don't all like the same things. Trust your own judgement and keep trying new classes until you experience the after class 'high' and you realise you didn't even check your watch once! The presenter's personality and communication style can make a big difference to your level of enjoyment.

IN A NUTSHELL:

- **Research** gym facilities, personal training and classes in your area. Extra knowledge will improve your confidence.

- **Ask a friend to join you** but don't delay if this is not an option. Develop courage to step out into *uncomfortable*.

- **Be open-minded to** finding out if the gym is an option for you. Arrange a free trial.

- **Investigate hiring a personal trainer.** Research options online and ask around for recommendations. Ask for a 'taster' trial session.

- **Try out new classes** and be armed with online information prior to attending so you know what to expect.

- **Look for positives** even if you decide the gym, training or classes are not suited to you. Be open-minded and keep exploring new options.

CHAPTER 5

Nourish to Flourish
Eating for wellness

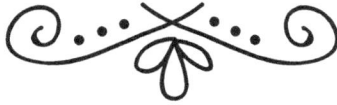

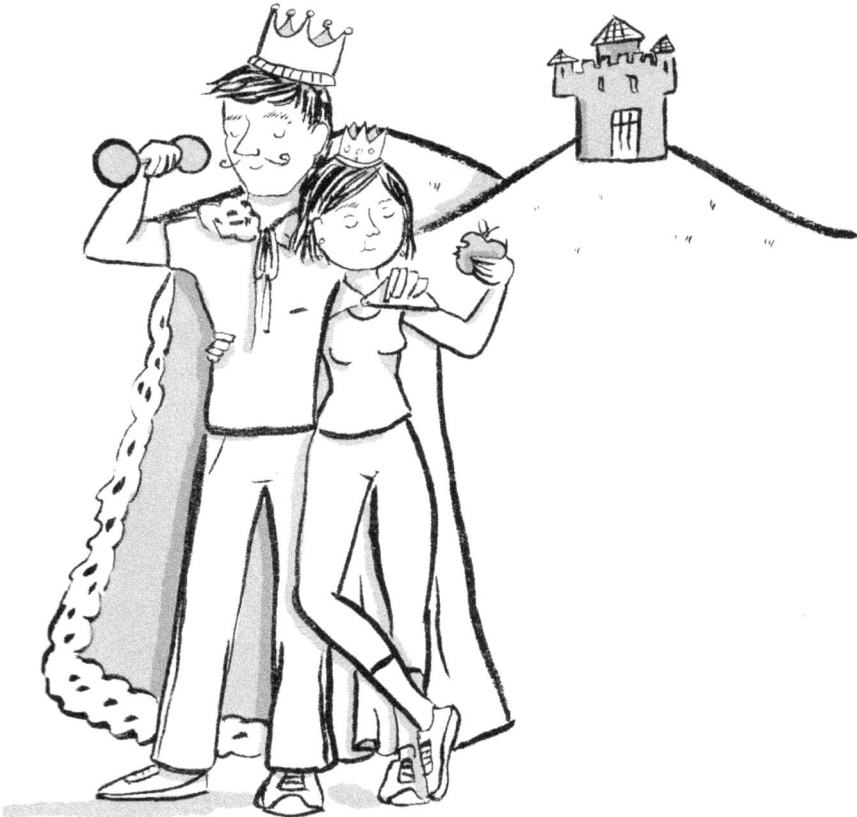

'Exercise is king. Nutrition is queen. Put them together and you've got a kingdom.'

– Jack LaLanne

Are you confused with an overload of info out there? Should I become *vegan*, try *intermittent fasting* or *the celebrity green banana peel diet?*

Many years ago, when wanting weight loss, I got sucked into eating copious amounts of soup on the Cabbage Soup diet! I also starved myself on powdered shakes in a desperate attempt to lose a few quick kilos before attending an ex-boyfriend's wedding! This is definitely *not* what I recommend you do! It's crazy that we can get drawn into such diet fads, but I can understand why they are so popular. When we want to shed some weight, it's tempting to want quick results and short-term commitments like 7 or 14 days. The fad plans are usually simple and we get told exactly what to do, plus we feel a surge of satisfaction when we actually see a shift on the scales, even if it is mainly fluid. They can *seem* to be good points ...

Whilst a quick detox can certainly give us a reboot and some good cleansing benefits, what about the fad plans? What happens afterwards? You need to know that the quick-fix fad plans can lead you into yo-yo dieting and long-term unhealthy relationships with food.

I too have scoured the supermarket shelves for the 'lite' or 'low cal' option whether it was warranted or not, marketed to us as somehow *healthier*. I'm not anti-diet plans or light options, but I can't help wondering how much better off we would be, with a *simple old-fashioned balanced approach to include most foods in moderation*, like it was before the wave of processed and convenience foods took over. The days when convenience foods were recognised as 'occasionals' rather than everyday mainstream.

I recall when soft drink, chips and lollies were reserved for parties, before they made their way into our pantries as an everyday entitlement. In the country town where I was raised, there was not a 'drive-through' in sight and a break from routine, consisted of fish and chips on a Friday night. Busy lives, laziness and being bombarded with clever marketing and diet trends, have contributed to this unhealthy culture that is fast becoming the new normal. Take a fresh look and realise that whilst it may not be as simple as the old days, the choice is still yours.

Free from fad

Long-term fresh healthy eating habits will give you freedom and a whole new relationship around food. When the emphasis is on eating mindfully with positivity and enjoyment, you will form a genuine desire to nourish and treat your body with the healthy respect it deserves.

Have you ever noticed that when you are told you *can't* have a desired food, you sometimes crave it even more? You might be successful at resisting it short term but if you do give in, it often leads to guilt and bingeing, further contributing to an unhealthy relationship around food.

Freedom—you be the boss!

Quit labelling foods as **good or bad!** It is far better to shift your mindset around food and stop categorising it in that way. Instead, lay it **ALL** on the table and trust yourself to choose with freedom, from an educated perspective and in line with your goals.

This means you could keep **ALL** foods in the options basket, but relegate some to the occasionals, very occasionals or not at all. Do so from an empowered position of knowing you *can* choose them, or choose to eliminate them if you want, based on an informed decision of how they make you feel or whether they align with your desired outcomes. Ask yourself, *'What can't I live without?'* and find a way to factor it in with moderation in mind. It can be managed with strategies such as portion size. If your *occasionals* start creeping into an everyday occurrence, then refer to Chapter 7 that deals with habits.

If weight loss is your goal and you prefer to follow a diet plan, then find one that guides you to focus on all the great options you **CAN** eat. Ditch rigid plans which include too many 'rules' on 'bad' foods or what you *shouldn't* eat as this can encourage a deprivation mindset and interfere with a positive outlook around food.

If someone deems chocolate cake to be 'bad' and eliminates it whilst trying to lose weight, in the future they may want a piece of cake at a party, but experience guilt for even a nibble. If, however, chocolate cake is considered an occasional, then there is far more freedom to choose.

This approach with moderation in mind, can set you up for life with a happy, positive association with food and have a flow-on effect for those around you. Choose a plan that focuses on the beautiful fresh healthy foods we are so fortunate to have access to in countries like Australia.

There has been an increase in anti-diet plans in recent times and the principles of **intuitive eating** are worth considering. Do your research and trust your own judgement to assess if this is for you. You can read up on topics like 'feel your fullness' and 'discover the satisfaction factor' on sites such as www.intuitiveeating.org.

Is the celebrity diet for me?

In Australia, personal trainers must act within their scope of practice. This means that I can provide general healthy eating information and advice in line with the Australian Dietary Guidelines, however I can't determine if that celebrity green banana peel diet is a match for you! Be mindful of following advice from your favourite celeb or influencer on Instagram and make up your own mind. If you require more specialised assistance, seek advice from a qualified professional in nutrition such as a registered practising dietitian, nutritionist or naturopath.

I found that those raging hormones of menopause were certainly calmed down with modifications to my diet along with herbs and other lifestyle tweaks. These were recommended by my naturopath and her guidance was invaluable. I also found *The Wisdom of Menopause* by Dr Christiane Northrup a good resource. I recall from her book that even some healthy foods were not advised for those experiencing menopausal symptoms. According to Chinese medicine, avoiding some heat-producing foods can help to relieve symptoms. I experienced a significant reduction in overheating by reducing alcohol consumption.

Vitamins and supplements

Once again, as a fitness professional, I cannot advise you on the suitability of supplementation. I do benefit from taking these occasionally as prescribed by a professional. Just because a supplement is chocolate flavoured with a funky label and the hot-looking salesperson selling them swears by them, they may not be the right fit for you. Do your own research.

What about probiotic and prebiotic supplementation? Antibiotics, chemical residues, certain foods you eat, and even stress can affect a healthy balance of gut bacteria. Before you rush out to buy supplements, find out about the many foods that can restore the balance naturally. *Why is it so important?* Research on **the gut-brain relationship** shows that healthy gut bacteria can play a role in everything from obesity, immunity and allergies, to mental health. We can increase our stock of good bacteria with probiotics, including cultured yoghurt and some fermented foods, and 'feed' the bacteria with prebiotics by eating certain types of dietary fibre—for example, asparagus and leeks.

Just hearing these facts might not inspire you to rush out now and stock up on sauerkraut, however you may change your mind after researching it further. Remember Giulia Enders? I mentioned her in Chapter 3, talking about how to sit on the toilet! Her book *Gut, the inside story to our body's most under-rated organ*, is uniquely different from other books I've read on the subject. Make it a priority to read, whether you have gut or bowel issues or not!

Benefits of good nutrition

Most of us are well informed on the importance of healthy eating habits and have experienced firsthand, the correlation between what we eat and how we feel. Some of those key benefits include:

- provides our bodies with the nutrients it needs to perform all its important functions—including fuel to skyrocket your jump squats!
- we will feel and look healthy and assist our immune system to function well
- assist in preventing disease and helping to manage health conditions including an imbalance of hormones and stress
- helps to maintain a healthy weight and improve our chance of a longer, better quality life.

If you don't have a healthy diet and regular physical activity, you could be at a higher risk of developing health problems such as heart disease, stroke, type 2 diabetes, cancer and other conditions like Alzheimer's disease. You can also miss out on feeling supercharged with energy.

Remember that disease does not appear overnight! There may be many years of unhealthy habits and lifestyle that has contributed.

According to the Australian Institute of Health and Welfare:

*'Chronic diseases feature more prominently among people **aged 45 and over**, while the leading causes of death among people aged 1–44 are external causes, such as accidents and suicides.*

In the period 2016–2018, the leading causes of death according to age were as follows: **Coronary heart disease was the leading cause of death for people aged 45–64,** *followed by lung cancer. For people aged 65–74, it was lung cancer followed by coronary heart disease. Dementia, including Alzheimer disease was the second leading cause of death among people aged 75 and older, behind coronary heart disease.'*

Take note of these statistics and don't become one of them!

When we already know we could do more to avoid becoming one of the statistics we've just read about, why DO we stuff rubbish down our throat and tell ourselves it's only a tiny morsel and it won't make a difference? I agree that an occasional chocolate binge is not the big issue here. It's the habits and things we do *every* day that make the difference. It's up to you to look carefully at the foods you consume and take into account the hidden elements such as sugar (often disguised with other names). I recommend watching *That sugar film* (2014) or read *That sugar guide* by Damon and Zoe Gameau. Our family watches the film once a year as a refresher and we all have a much greater awareness of the impact it has on our health *and* our teeth!

The cupcake inequity effect

Some years ago, whilst attending a seminar, I learned that weight loss was much more than a calorie in calorie out approach, and other influences could affect results such as medications, hormones, stress and fatigue. After delving deeper into research, I once again tuned into a seminar presented by Dr Cam McDonald, whom I referred to earlier in relation to behavioural change.

Dr Cam drew on his professional experience in his dietitian practice and talked about the *cupcake inequity effect,* where some people can eat one cupcake and seem like they gain three kilos whilst another person can eat the same cake and seem to *lose* weight! He said, 'One man's food is another man's poison'.

Through the use of examples of the variance of information on the same food, Dr Cam said, *'I could pluck out two different articles with studies on red meat. One will refer to the negative effects of eating red meat such as higher risk of colorectal cancer or heart disease. Another article may discuss the benefits of the quality protein assisting in body composition. Which article do we listen to? No wonder there is confusion!'*

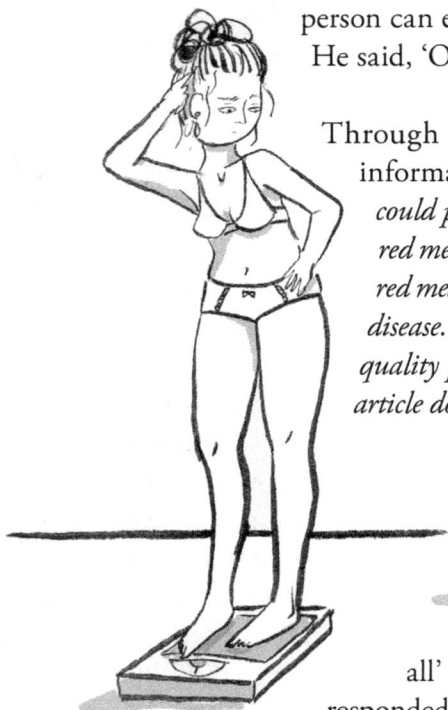

One size does not fit all

I have never liked a 'one size fits all' approach. I have observed how clients have responded differently to the same food and exercise programs. There are many out there who make great choices but don't get the results they are after: the non-responders. This can be very demotivating when someone else they know is following the exact same plan and will get the results they expected. Why?

Dr Cam explained how a personalised approach incorporating epigenetics, can determine what to do based on our unique suitability for certain foods and exercise. It takes into account scientific based theories and solutions to account for our genetic make-up, unique body design and other factors. Even how we interact socially and deal with stress can affect how our foods are metabolised as well as the timing of when we eat, based on the science of chronobiology.

If you are seemingly doing and eating all the right things, yet not getting the desired results, then learning more about this scientific approach could be the answer.

Dr Cam's science-based explanation whet my appetite (pardon the pun) to take up further studies in the area of personalised health incorporating epigenetics. I am currently studying this area of health and its impact, to help clients further with all aspects of their wellness. If you would like to know more about this scientific approach, please subscribe to the link on my website. Visit: www.reclaimingyou.com.au.

Accordingly, I will not set out specific nutritional advice in this chapter and I won't be advising you on how many red apples to eat in a day or whether you should cut out red meat! It needs to be tailored for you and I can help you with this once I know more about YOU! However, I have set out my simple eating for wellness tips and these are given with caution of *one size does not fit all*—take on board what works for **you**.

1. GET INSPIRED

Mix it up with variety—make it social and fun
It can be easy to get into a rut and prepare the same meals over and over. To mix things up, try out some or all of the following ideas:

Find inspiration to learn. Stay fresh and motivated by thumbing through magazines, books, websites, attending workshops, listening to podcasts and watching cooking shows.

Try something new. Aim to introduce one new healthy food or recipe every week and be adventurous with weekend breakfasts to step out of your weekday routine. You can also try new ways of cooking by enrolling in a cooking class, in person or online.

GYO. Experiment with Growing Your Own food, starting small with fresh herbs, lettuce or tomatoes. It is so satisfying to eat something fresh from your own garden. If you are short on space, a small herb planter box near the kitchen works well or convert an old wheelbarrow into an edible garden on wheels.

Another option is to sprout your own seeds, grains and beans which can be grown in jam jars in a matter of days. I experimented with sprouting many years ago when I was out at sea for several months with little access to fresh produce. Sprouts have a high nutritional value and are a fresh living food. You can add them to salads and soups, roll them in a leaf of lettuce or crunch them as nibbles.

Get others involved. Trade recipes or meals with friends or have a competition to encourage variety and more of a social element. During the COVID-19 isolation at my house, we introduced a theme-based cooking competition. We all cooked one special meal a week each, which was fun and tasty, particularly the Mexican theme when I managed to give my sombrero another airing!

Challenge yourself. Add further challenge to food-based competitions such as eliminating or adding something out of a diet for 30 days.

Be creative. Unleash your creativity and experiment with juices and smoothies. They are also a great opportunity to sneak more vegies into your diet. Try to incorporate more vegetables than fruit in your drinks to lower the sugar content. Smoothies can be substantial when they have a protein base such as almond milk and be satisfying as an alternative light meal option. Play with colour by adding a variety of vegetables on your plate to make it look enticing. Use garnishes of fresh herbs, edible flowers or a slice of orange or strawberry for that finishing touch.

Choosing a plan
Your personality type and circumstances can influence whether you prefer a fixed dietary plan to follow or an unstructured approach.

Some people find that an 80/20 plan works well (or 70/30) of eating mainly fresh, unprocessed food for 80 per cent of the time whilst the other 20 per cent allows for those 'occasionals' and Friday night fish n chips! Aiming for 100 per cent 'perfect' eating, can set people up for failure or lead to a stressful obsession, which is not good for digestion either.

If you follow a structured plan, ensure it suits **your** body. For example, the intermittent fasting diet may be better suited for those bodies whose digestive system is good at conserving and storing energy, such that they can function well by not eating for several hours. Compare this to another person who digests food quickly and needs to eat every three to four hours to avoid blood sugar level slumps and grumps. *How will you know?* Trialling a diet will give you some indication of its suitability, based on how you feel physically and mentally, or run it past an expert. You could also have a personalised health assessment to help determine that suitability.

A word on detox

I'm often asked about detox and whether it is a good idea. Consider your personal reasons for doing so to determine what method will work best. Options range from elimination of various foods and stimulants through to extreme juice fasting. Consult a qualified professional to assess what is right for you.

Personally, I like to do a simple detox once a year for 5–7 days for the following benefits:

- it resets my tastebuds and helps to reduce sugar cravings
- it allows me to re-evaluate any unwanted habits that have crept into my diet, like exceeding my daily quota of coffees!
- I enjoy becoming reacquainted with some delicious herbal teas
- it gives me a boost, feeling lighter, refreshed and energised
- after the detox, I'm highly motivated to make healthier choices and am more discerning about what I let back into my diet!

My own short-term detox involves cutting out processed foods, sugar and stimulants like caffeine and alcohol, reducing or eliminating dairy products and basing my meals around lots of fruit and vegetables with lean protein. I incorporate some carbohydrates to satisfy my energy requirements at the time. During the detox, I drink only water and herbal teas. If I suffer withdrawal symptoms or get hungry, tired or grumpy, I manage it by drinking a cup of thick pureed vegetable soup.

Create your own guide

Create dietary guidelines for your household, which may constitute a plan around Friday night takeaway or certain foods that you don't want to be brought into your home. At my house, we have zero tolerance on MSG and if something sneaks through in a disguised format, it goes straight into the rubbish bin!

If you live with others, create a plan together and you'll have more buy-in. If you have kids, let them know that you want to improve your own health and how that will translate to real benefits to them.

'But Mum, please can we have those choc chip muffins included in our plan?'

'Yep, sure—but we are going to store them in the freezer in a non-see-through container (I'm good at forgetting what I can't see) *and how about you have them twice a week at the time of your choosing? No, not before breakfast! Oh, and by the way, with this new healthy eating plan, I'm going to have a ton of energy real soon, so instead of dropping you off for rock climbing, I'm coming WITH you—see you at the top! Anyway kids, let's have a bake-off competition for the best choc chip beetroot muffins.'*

Calorie/kilojoule counting

I'm not a fan of calorie counting however it can be helpful to have some knowledge about the calorie count of food and drinks, to bring awareness to substitutions that may work better and help with portion size. For example, 250ml lemonade (approximately 108 calories) vs. mineral water with fresh lime or lemon (approximately 6 calories).

Once you have awareness, counting calories is NOT a good long-term strategy unless you've been advised by a health professional, such as to help manage a medical condition. It can become obsessive and place too much focus on every morsel that goes in your mouth, so keep it casual once you become more familiar.

Understanding the difference in the nutritional value in foods is important. While two foods may have the same calorie count, there can be a huge disparity in the portion size and nutritional value. It is interesting to compare foods in this way and it will have more impact if you visually see the two items side by side. There are many websites that demonstrate this well. For example, according to the ZME Science website: *'a chocolate bar can pack more calories than one kilogram of vegetables.'* If you recognise the nutritional value of both from a position of awareness, yet *still* want the chocolate, then go for it!

Keeping a food diary can be valuable to examine the correlation between foods eaten and how you feel. It can also be helpful to show to a nutritional coach to learn more about your eating habits. As with calorie counting, ensure that keeping a food diary does not turn into a chore or an obsession, and you have a valid short-term reason to do so.

2. GET ORGANISED

Now it's time to get organised …

Clean out the pantry and fridge

Cleaning out the pantry is not one of my favourite jobs, so I like to get it over with quickly, but thoroughly. When I do so, I'm a woman on a mission frantically unpacking copious amounts of baked beans to the kitchen bench—a touch of COVID-19 panic buying evident. I like to do this to fast, funky music with the timer urging me on!

Here's an outline of my approach:

- *Everything* must come out of the pantry (Marie Kondo style). Okay, it may take longer than the one hour you set aside. Think about asking someone to step in and help, even booking a cleaning agency for a few hours. Students may be enthusiastic where money is involved. And whilst you've got that help, clean out your fridge as well.

- Ditch the 'out of dates' and any rubbish items that contain unhealthy additives. I refer to my *Additive Alert Book* by Julie Eady to remind me why I hate E621 and the cheeky way they try and call it a flavour *enhancer*. Puleeeeease!

- Treats—fair enough. Not everyone in the household wants to give up chocolate Tim Tams, but hopefully, you have agreed with others in your family, that these are to be occasionals. I do have some of these items in my pantry and they live in a brown paper bag at the back of a deep cupboard. They require a ladder to access them. Perfect. The last time we had to bring the ladder out, involved a fun, quirky, taste testing game for some international visitors. More often than not, in my annual Kondo clean up next year, I will find those brown paper bags still intact and even out of date. Yessss! Far better to give them away even to the bin than clogging up my arteries.

Restock shopping

Just a reminder: DO NOT go shopping before you've eaten. Your resolve may be weakened when you are tempted at the promo trolley in the supermarket aisle to try the yummy little bite-size things hanging off toothpicks. Hot and salted off the portable grill in-store, they are usually delicious. The morsel itself is not the problem. I have ended up buying the product only to get home and realise *why* it tasted so good. Shame I didn't have my glasses on in the shop. Ditch. Those pesky

E numbers again! Another reason to clean your teeth before going shopping too. Those morsels will not mix well with mint toothpaste.

Shop with a list—and stick to it. If you struggle with temptation at the shops, then do an online order and remember to add 'brown paper bags'.

Where possible, try and support your local greengrocer or farmers' market. The produce will be fresher, as a lot of the fruit and vegetables in supermarkets have been in cold storage for a long time, which means the nutrient value (and taste) can be compromised. Wash fruit and vegetables well at home, and if it is within your budget, consider home grown or organic produce to avoid harmful chemicals.

Get cooking, get organised

Aim to prepare as much of your own food as possible. You would be amazed at the hidden fats, salts, sugars and MSG in some restaurant and café food that make it taste so yummy. Minimise the use of packaged sauces (often full of additives) and scan the labels to ensure you know exactly what you are putting into your body.

Some people control portion size by using smaller plates ... I wonder if they ever feel deprived. For me, bread and butter size just won't cut it! I prefer to use normal size dinner plates but trick the brain by filling it up mostly with a beautiful colourful salad or vegies *first*, then add on the rest. If you tend to overeat spaghetti or rice-based meals from a bowl, use the dinner plate trick too.

My friends know about my love for vegie soup and I always have a freezer full of containers of my special blend. It will reduce your hunger whilst you are cooking, or you can supplement the soup with some plates of other bits and pieces for an easy Sunday night supper. If my family want occasional 'junk food', then they need to balance it out with an entrée of my famous soup.

These are some of the other simple ways I set myself up for healthy eating:

- Have a weekly or fortnightly cook-up and stock up the freezer with some nutritious meals or soup. It's handy to have some options on standby for those nights when you are short on time.

- For lunch on the go, prep items in advance. If you prep in the morning or the night before, you won't be as tempted to reach for a quick junky option on the fly.

- Same goes for prepping snacks into containers for when the munchies strike. Expand on the carrot and celery staples and get creative with a wide variety of vegies and fruit. Use clear containers to store them, which will encourage you to see them first when you open the fridge—beckoning you with their beautiful assortment of colours.

3. EATING OUT

Cafés and eateries

When you head out for a meal, if you get to choose the venue and don't want to overeat, stay away from buffets unless you have strong willpower, or it is an occasional thing. Too much temptation for me! If I'm doing a buffet, then breakfast is the best option.

If you find yourself struggling to see something on the menu to fit into your healthy eating plan, don't be shy in asking staff to cook something that's not on the menu or opt for a grilled version. If you don't want the deep-fried fillers, ask for extra vegies or salad instead, and request sauces to be served on the side. Your friends will wish they did the same. *'That looks sensational—I didn't see THAT on the menu!'*

Drinks and functions

If you plan on drinking alcohol or sugary drinks when out, decide in advance what you would like to consume and then find tricks to support your decision. In BYO situations, don't take more than you want to consume. Alternatively, be generous and share your wine with everyone at the table. You can also volunteer to be the driver. No alcohol then.

If you're attending a function, take the edge off your appetite before you arrive. This could mean eating a small bowl of soup, or something else nutritious and light to help curb your hunger and balance out those canapés and spring rolls.

At home, use the brown paper bag strategy for wine as well. It might just need a little chilling first, but is better than the suggestive temptation staring you in the face when opening the fridge. *Pick me, pick me!* The tiny mini bottles hit the spot if you only want one glass when on your own ... super expensive, often pricier than the full 750ml however they can assist to prevent that conversation that goes, '*The wine is already open—may as well finish it off and not waste it.*'

Here are some more ideas to limit your alcohol intake:

- avoid having your glass topped up—you are in control and can decide how many glasses are enough
- be mindful of what you drink in relation to your wellness goals—if it is weight loss, choose carefully and consider the high sugar content in bubbly
- dilute your wine with ice-cubes or have a wine spritzer with soda water—less alcohol, less sugar
- drink sparkling water in a wine glass when out and you will not be pressured by others to join them.

Q&A

Q. What if I'm cutting down on sugar and my family are not interested in doing so too?

Don't nag them and instead of trying to convert or police others, just do it yourself and allow them to witness your changes through your example. They may be inspired to do it in their own time.

Q. What if I know I need to drink more water but often get busy and forget?

Always carry a water bottle when you go out. Set up a reminder on your phone or try a hydration app that tracks your intake and reminds you when it's time to drink up. If your phone is paired to a watch, even better to receive that prompt with a vibrational jolt!

Q. I am finding it hard to lose weight even though I eat healthy meals. I've heard that I need to change my food routine of what and when I eat. What does this mean?

If you've been stuck on repeat mode, following the same menu plan every day, you've been helping to keep your weight stable! Wake up your digestive system and mix things up with variety. Start by substituting breakfast with a new choice. Epigenetics and the science of chronobiology can help you understand that the timing of when you eat can also affect your body's response to nutrition and digestion.

IN A NUTSHELL:

10 Tips for successful eating for wellness

1. Try one new recipe or food every week. That's 52 over a year!

2. Get organised—spruce up your pantry and fridge with a makeover.

3. Prepare some meals and snacks in advance and be ready for when the munchies strike.

4. Drink water half to one hour before eating and minimise drinking throughout the meal as it can interfere with digestive juices.

5. Create your ideal environment for calm and comfort at mealtimes, and when practical, eat at a time that suits your body.

6. Practise eating mindfully, chewing food well and slowing down.

7. Enjoy the social aspect of food with great conversation.

8. Practise gratitude for your body and enjoy nourishing it with a beautiful variety of colourful fresh food including lots of vegetables and fruit. Focus on all the great foods you CAN eat that make you feel good.

9. Practise freedom of choice and change your internal dialogue of labelling foods as good or bad—manage your choices through education and awareness in line with your desired outcomes.

10. Keep learning to stay fresh and informed. Investigate the principles of intuitive eating. Try a personalised health assessment for specific recommendations tailored for you.

CHAPTER 6

SPARK Goals
Plan for your vision to come true

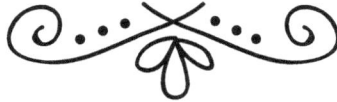

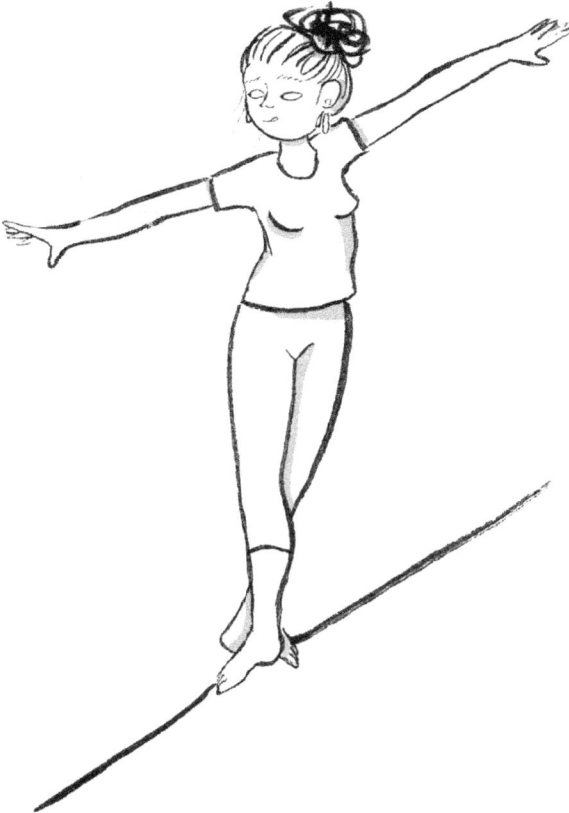

'A goal should scare you a little and excite you
a lot.'

- Joe Vitale

Have you ever set the *same or similar* health goals on New Year's Day, for several years running? I've done it too—sometimes they worked and other times they fizzled out around March. Before long, I would feel like I was in *Groundhog Day,* sitting there on January 1, setting the same goal over and over, losing count of how many consecutive years in a row.

There are many reasons for failed attempts, and this chapter will focus on how to set goals in a way that sets you up for success.

Goal setting is a vital element of bringing your vision to life. Your personal health goals will have power and meaning if they are chosen with your wellness vision clearly in mind. Goals give you a tailored personalised plan like having a map to guide positive change in the most efficient way. For some, this may be achieving a goal using a fast, direct route whilst for others, it could be an intentional slower explorative journey to bring about that change. YOU get to choose.

Regardless of the timeframe, one of the most important elements of goal setting is to determine what small steps need to be taken and plan how they will be achieved. If you don't back up your goals by developing an action plan, you may experience an unintentional slow meandering journey with a loss of focus, a failed attempt, or it might be another quick fix.

We live in a world of quick fixes and promises, boasting enticing results in record time. This is not *always* a bad thing and can be an exciting lure to at least get us off the couch. If we believe that something will take forever, we can lose interest. But this goal-driven focus can have its negatives too. If you *do* want fast results but are also receptive to the possibilities of long-term change, you will need to learn how to plan and enjoy your journey. This includes breaking goals down into small manageable steps.

There has been a shift in thinking over recent years that we can be too focused on the end results of achieving goals, rather than the journey getting there. When our impatience drives us to want immediate results through goal-driven focus, we can feel pressured and have unrealistic fantasies that can leave us in a state of inaction and disappointment. We might have short-term success but in the long run, can have a 'yo-yo' experience which can chip away at our confidence and self-esteem.

Kaizen

Kaizen is a Japanese philosophy of continuous improvement of working practices and personal efficiency. It comes from the words 'kai' meaning 'change' and 'zen' meaning 'good'. Kaizen can lead to consistent long-term changes in behaviours and habits. It is a concept that has proved successful for many corporations, sporting teams and individuals. It involves developing consistent everyday actions to build habits for continuous improvement.

Try a Kaizen-inspired approach of planning a system of breaking goals down into small manageable chunks, with a sustainable series of tasks to support them. Focus on progression and improvement by adopting a mindset of saying, *'What can I do today to take me closer to my vision?' and 'What are the daily or weekly behaviours or habits that will help me achieve my goal?'*

This is how Rock Star Suzi used a series of everyday actions for continual improvement to achieve mini goals and achieve long-term benefits.

We started small and chose a few goals. Suzi wanted to increase her energy and develop strength and stamina for stage performances. She wanted to lose 5kg, develop social confidence and come to the gym 2–3 times per week on her own. This was currently way outside her comfort zone. She suffered extreme shyness, lack of confidence and didn't know one piece of gym equipment from another.

We reduced Suzi's fitness goal to a mini goal of twice-weekly personal training sessions to learn about strength training methods and how to use the equipment. We also prioritised her goal of social confidence so that she could practise coming to the gym on her own. We set up weekly mini goals and a series of actions that she could work on daily.

We did not focus on the weight loss goal yet, as her new planned behaviours would assist in achieving this with little effort. Instead, she planned to introduce one new dietary substitution every week (or two weeks, depending on how she managed), starting with swapping Coke for water. Once she blitzed that, she would move on to the next swap. She would add in a plan to get in more daily incidental activity in a similar way.

Her action plan for social confidence, started with simple interaction at the gym with a nod or smile to the person on the reception desk. We kept raising the bar to look for daily opportunities to take her closer to her goal of confidently engaging in social conversation, and before long, she had graduated to approaching total strangers to talk about workout plans. This progressive approach took the pressure off worrying about how to achieve the larger goal as she got to celebrate successful actions every day.

Your vision comes to life

This chapter will focus on bringing your vision to life to move you closer to living the optimal healthy life you desire. We will discuss some tips to help you set goals as well as the supporting strategies that go alongside them to maximise their success.

Before we start, let's take a bird's-eye view of the steps involved in this method of goal planning:

- develop confidence
- review your wellness vision
- set some goals (1–3 to start with)

- chunk goals down into mini goals
- reduce them down to regular actionable steps.

I have given you some tips below to help support this process. Just a word of warning: keep it simple and don't over-plan or set too many goals. Start small and chip away.

I want you to consider goal setting in a *sparky* way with enthusiasm and passion. Many people use a formal system of SMART goals. In keeping this simple and fun, lets change the SMART to SPARK and call these your **SPARK GOALS!** I want words like Spark, Passion and Action to generate feelings of excitement and remind you **why** you are doing this. As you set goals around your wellness, *Feel the Spark and Passion to fuel the Actions to get Results and stay Keen.*

1. DEVELOP CONFIDENCE

Step outside of fear to uncomfortable

Do you have any resistance around goal setting? People can sometimes show resistance to goal setting because deep down they fear failure and accountability. *Hey—if I don't set a goal, then I won't have to fail at it, and if I don't tell anyone about it and don't achieve it, then no-one will even know that I've failed … I might just stay comfortable.*

When trying to overcome fear, it is natural to feel slightly *uncomfortable*. After all, we have a natural tendency to move towards pleasure (often short term) rather than pain. You may have chosen a goal around increasing your walking fitness and decided on a new regime of early morning walks. Staying in a warm snug bed at 6 am when the alarm goes off, can have us wanting to snuggle up for another round or more of snooze. Staying in bed seems to be the more pleasurable option. The pain of getting out of bed when you really don't feel like it, is the slightly uncomfortable option.

Jumping out of bed and putting on your runners, becomes a whole lot more meaningful if we are looking at the big picture, and know that the *uncomfortable* is an action that will take you closer to achieving your goal and realising your vision.

It will become easier each day and you could look for signs that it is becoming that way. *I got out of bed easier this morning and only hit the snooze button once. I feel proud of myself for rising (literally) to the challenge.* Tell yourself that it is getting easier each day until your brain believes it and suddenly one day, you will be almost out the door with your runners on wondering how that even happened!

Overcoming obstacles

Face any fears you have around setting goals and keep them in perspective. Ask yourself what could I do to become more confident around setting and achieving them? Look at your own set of strengths and then what obstacles could get in the way. Your strength might be that you're determined and like to try new things like enjoying a sunrise walk. On the other side of the coin, perhaps you don't have confidence that you will be able to get up early in the morning. *You've never been a 'morning' person.*

Look for solutions to overcome your obstacle, such as asking a buddy to meet you for the walk. Bear in mind, that particular goal may need tweaking. It may have been unrealistic to plan to get up early every single day and so you might start with trying it once per week and grow confidence (baby steps). You might also adapt your goal of daily walks by swapping sunrise for sunset, which could be more enjoyable and achievable for YOU.

Set yourself up for success and don't model your goals on the goals of other people. These are YOUR goals! Try to problem-solve possible solutions to overcome all obstacles that could get in the way. *What if ... happens? Then I will ...*

2. TIPS WHEN SETTING YOUR GOALS

Don't try and change everything at once. Focus on what you know is achievable and mildly challenging too.

Avoid overwhelm: If you focus on all the things you would need to do over the next few months, it can feel daunting and totally overwhelming. Practise success with mini goals and actionable steps to develop new behaviours and habits. If we obsess and take too much on too quickly or if progress doesn't match up, we can feel stressed and can experience a sense of failure.

Keep it simple: Some people already LOVE setting goals. Congrats! If this is not you, don't worry. Goal setting does not have to be a bore or a chore. This is NOT a business goal setting exercise. These are your **SPARK goals!**

Write them down: Write your goals down in a diary or journal so they are clear and focused with your vision in mind. Choose goals that are easy to start with and that you are excited about achieving. If you are unsure, you could choose one goal around **exercise**, one for **healthy eating** and one for **relaxation**.

Time frame: You can choose a time frame that suits your goal and vision—this could be one year, six months, three months, one month or weekly goals. No matter the time frame, it must be backed up with small manageable actions to get you there. If you are creating a goal around fitness, then three months is a reasonable time, where changes are usually significant. From there, write down mini goals and daily steps to help you achieve the goal and grow new long-term habits.

Baby steps—daily action plan: When breaking down the goals, think of the smallest version you can reduce it to and start there. Decide *'What small action can I do today to bring me closer to my goal* *of …'* Write these in your diary too. It is satisfying and motivating to tick off those daily achievements of success.

Practise success with chunking—one day at a time: Here's an example using a one-day approach:

At the gym, 52-year-old Bella asked a common question: 'How do I give up alcohol?' We talked about why it was important to her and the benefits she wanted. The thought of setting a goal of giving up alcohol for even a month seemed out of the realms of possibility, so it was easier to not even start. After more discussion, we renegotiated her goal to be more realistic and broke it down into mini goals. Her new goal was to break the daily habit and to enjoy alcohol on weekends with dinner or special occasions.

*Bella wasn't entirely confident, but I said, 'Can you get through **one** day like today, and substitute your alcohol with mineral water infused with fresh lime?' 'Oh sure, today would be easy as I don't usually drink on Mondays unless netball finishes early …'. I suggested she write it down in her diary and place a tick or a symbol for her daily success.*

After feeling proud of three days in a row with no alcohol, Bella decided to see how many 'one days' she could clock up in the week. Each day became easier to say no, especially as she began to experience better sleep. She was feeling good and proud of herself for achieving lots of 'one day' success.

Bella found it easier to turn this into new weekly goals and a monthly goal. She had developed the confidence to say 'I've nailed it. I'm good at it. I get to choose and design what I want, which is to enjoy alcohol on the weekends and special occasions.' After developing that confidence, Bella started on a new nutritional goal starting with the one-day approach.

Being successful in this way brings confidence and great aha *'Oh what a feeling!'* moments with big high five Toyota jumps! There is a neurochemical process in your brain that says, *'You rock at this, do more of it!'*. Celebrate it and before long, other goals will seem much more achievable.

Practise success. One day at a time. Can you challenge yourself to a week? A month? A year? This is the way to develop new habits.

Enjoy the journey: Place more emphasis on the enjoyment of success that comes with small regular actions that are leading to your goal. This takes the pressure off failing at the goal. Yes, that goal is still in sight, but we are also enjoying the ride and the everyday success of our achievements.

Consistency: Do what you can every day and adapt, even if that means working on your goal for only a few minutes. Be consistent! Do that without beating yourself up with negativity. Instead, pride yourself on the fact that you are moving towards your goal.

Learning opportunities: If you struggle on a particular day, then view it as a learning opportunity rather than a setback. It is not a failure. You may benefit from further support in helping you develop new strategies to support your desired changes.

Cut yourself some slack: Keep in mind the 80/20 or 70/30 rule. You don't need to be 'perfect' all the time. You are human!

3. TIPS TO SUPPORT YOUR GOALS

Allow that vision and goal to keep lighting up your path but live more in the present by focusing on the actionable steps right in front of you. Keep looking for those opportunities to celebrate daily. Remember, goals are great for planning your journey and systems are good for making progress.

So, now you have your goals, here are a few more tips to keep you on track.

- **Be flexible:** As you gain confidence, keep learning and questioning new challenges under the wellness vision umbrella. Be prepared for flexibility. A goal that you've set may not be as appealing as first thought, or the focus can change.

  I've had clients who had weight loss goals and we put in place manageable small actions to take them closer to their goal. Sometimes along the way, they realise (just like I did all those years ago), that they were enjoying the process of being active on their journey and that goal was no longer as important. Keep reviewing your vision and goals and stay flexible.

- **Accountability:** Create a new habit of reviewing your goals and actions on the same day and time every week. Sunday evenings work well for me. Review the past week and reflect on how you went and anything you learned that could help you in the future. Then plan tasks for the week ahead.

- **Social support:** Sharing your goals can strengthen your commitment and help with accountability. If you have a support team on board, they can encourage and help you to troubleshoot as well as celebrate.

- **Rewards:** Celebrate and bask in pride but don't stop there. Keep moving towards your next challenge on the wellness journey and set new goals.

  Rewards can be the benefits you are feeling and the sense of satisfaction from everyday improvement. You might also choose to reward yourself with treats that are related to your health. Things like a massage, new gym shoes or a foam roller!

Q&A

Q. What if I get sick and can't achieve my weekly tasks?
Resume when you can. If you can't manage what you had planned, adapt and take some tiny, small action, even if it is only for a few minutes. This action could be researching or journaling.

Q. What if I don't set goals because I already know what I need to do?
Knowing and doing are two different things. Planning will ensure you stay on track and will remind and reinforce you of the small tasks to do that form part of that goal.

Q. I've tried setting goals before and lost interest after a while.
Perhaps the goals were unrealistic or not meaningful. Ensure you have invested time to set up your personal wellness vision to provide focus and inspiration for your goals.

IN A NUTSHELL:

- **Develop confidence**. Address any fears.
- **Develop your plan** and write it down.
- **Review** your wellness vision.
- **Set some goals** (1–3 to start with).
- **Chunk goals down** into mini goals.
- **Reduce them** down to regular actionable steps.
- **Develop accountability** and support.
- **Make a plan** to overcome obstacles.
- **Celebrate** daily success!

CHAPTER 7

The Good, the Bad and the Better
Our habits and associations

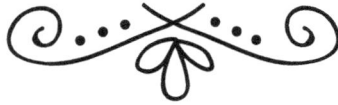

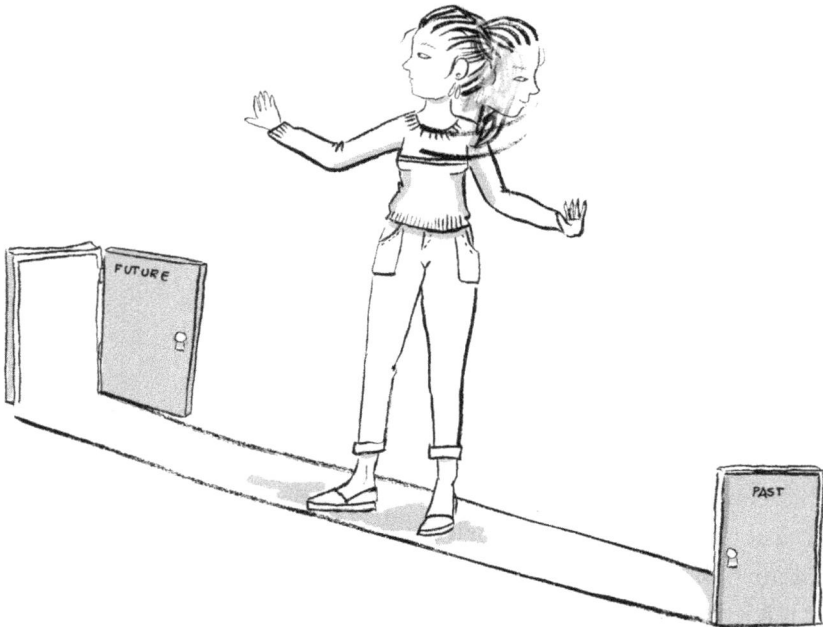

'Every time you are tempted to react in the same old way, ask if you want to be a prisoner of the past or a pioneer of the future.'

– Deepak Chopra

Habits can get a bad rap—but they can be a fantastic way to free ourselves from making a zillion decisions about everything we need to do. We get to give our brain a break and do things without much effort or decision-making. When you pop your seatbelt on, you don't need to wonder whether or not it's a good idea. It is a habit which seems to happen automatically.

But sometimes, habits can lead us astray …

Habits can tempt us with easy options and familiarity that prove resistant to change. Such sticky well-established habits can lead us on a merry dance, reinforcing behaviour that doesn't sit well with our healthy vision and goals.

If we don't make a concerted effort to change those habits, they will stay comfortably in repeat mode clocking up repetitions until they graduate to autopilot status. Once there, they are even more stubborn and hard to change! Firm action is required to take back control and set about changing them.

It's a deal!

It's up to you to decide which habits you deem 'good' and which to change. These may constitute behaviours that you prefer to be occasional. For example, chocolate is not bad, but you may consider a daily habit of having it for breakfast an undesirable habit. For ease of reference, let's refer to those **habits** as 'the Baddies'.

Imagine you are playing a Game of Habits—*the Good, the Bad and the Better*! The goal is to end up with a hand of cards that best support your goal. Discard *the Baddies* or use cunning and smart game strategies to trade them for *the Betters*. Hold on tightly to *the Good*—they are definite keepers, just like the ace!

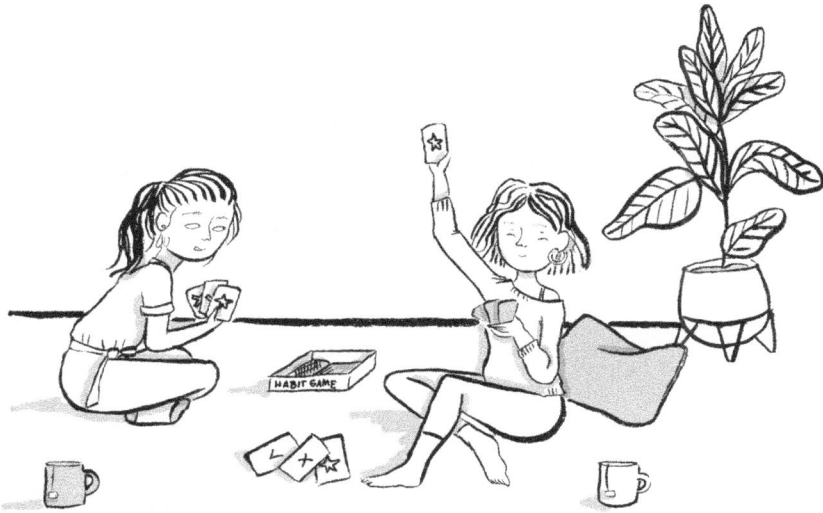

The Good

So now you have your winning hand, let's look at how do we build those good habits into part of our daily life that we can sustain long term? How can we elevate them to auto status? How do we do so without the mental chatter of *'Will I or won't I hit the snooze button?'* The way to do that is by *repetition*.

Repeat ... repeat ... and repeat some more ...

You may have experienced a hint of this when automatically using the indicators in your car to turn left or right. If you then jump into an unfamiliar European vehicle and don't consciously remind yourself, you will put the windscreen wipers on every time you turn the corner. Conscious behaviour will fix this until repetition helps the new habit kick in.

Take another example of running in the morning. It can be hard going in the beginning, but if you keep doing it regularly and for long enough, it will become easy. Because you've already made the commitment and your clothes and shoes are all laid out beside you, it can seem that you hardly remember consciously how you even came to be outside running and breathing in the fresh air. It is such a great feeling when our desired behaviours turn into reliable habits and feel effortless.

'Motivation is what gets you started. Habit is what keeps you going.'

– Jim Ryun

In my 20s, I shared a house with Greg, and I quizzed him one day about his great fitness habits. He said: *'I don't have to think about whether to do it or not. I've already decided that I like to go for a run every day. My body is programmed to head out the door at 5pm, without even realising how I get there. I just do it.'* I realise now, it was that determination and discipline to build a repetitive behaviour that got him started, until habits kicked in to set off his internal alarm clock at 4.55pm to get his trainers on. Nice one Greg!

How long does it take?

You may be wondering how long it takes to reinforce a habit? It depends on which study your read and what the habit is. Unplugging from technology one hour before bed may be easier and quicker to build a new habit around than an early morning run. It is tempting to want the fastest and easiest path. I have often been seduced by clever marketing that promises to change a habit in 21 days! That timeframe is a great *start* ...

There are many theories you will hear with magic formulas—three weeks, three months, three years ... It will take as long as it takes!

Take it a day at a time and remember the Kaizen model of continuous improvement. No matter how long it takes to become easy or auto, keep looking for those winning signs that it is becoming easier every day. You will find the process more enjoyable as you celebrate that daily success.

This leads us to the great sense of satisfaction we have, when we develop good habits that make it easy to achieve our goals. Habits are the workhorses that go about influencing the success of our goals.

'To change a habit, you must keep the old cue and deliver the old reward, but insert a new routine.'
– Charles Duhigg

In an online presentation, I heard Charles Duhigg explain how habits work. He talked about the three main parts: a cue or trigger, the routine (the habit stemming from behaviour) and a reward. The reward is how our neurology learns to encode this pattern for the future and the effect they have on actions—consciously or not.

As I researched more about habits, I realised just how much there is to learn, and it could take me years! Rather than regurgitate information from the pros, I will leave it to you to hear it from the experts in behavioural science. I have simply shared my own strategies that have helped my clients and me; feel free to see if they can work for you too. If you do want to understand more about the science behind habits and behaviour change, then get it from the horse's mouth. I enjoyed reading *Atomic Habits* by James Clear and an easy to read practical guide called *The How of Habits* by Bri Williams.

1. DEVELOP AWARENESS OF BEHAVIOUR

Conscious choice or habit?

Do your unwanted behaviours stem from conscious choice or are they part of a habit? If they are coming from a habit, then boot them out and toss them onto the *discard* pile! If you are choosing the behaviour consciously (or you *think* you are), then some delay tactics can help.

Delay tactics

Here's an example of one of Bella's strategies …

You may recall that Bella was trying to limit her wine consumption to weekends only. So here it is Wednesday, and she feels like a glass of wine … no huge burning desire or need, just a mild craving for it. Before rummaging through the cupboard to retrieve the brown paper-bagged bottle, she gives herself the 'OK' to have it, on the proviso that she waits half an hour. She wants to know: 'Do I really want it? Or is it just a passing craving?' In the meantime, she gets busy (with activity). If, after half an hour, she's not taken her eye off the clock and is salivating in anticipation, then she enjoys that one glass or two, happy with her conscious awareness of choice.

Sometimes, she's noticed that by waiting half an hour and getting immersed in activity, she loses track of time and realises that the craving has passed.

2. HOW TO MANAGE 'THE BADDIES'

Replace, wean or cold turkey?

As a reminder, 'the Baddies' is only a term I've used to describe the undesirable **HABIT**, *not* the actual food or behaviour.

Replace it

Replace the Baddies with something similar but healthier ('the Better'). For example, *I'm going to replace my daily glass of sugary juice with a glass of sparkling mineral water with fresh lime'. 'Swap milky cappuccino for long black or herbal'.* **What the?!!!** Yessss, I know it is easier said than done if the thought of a cuppa without milk makes you cringe! It doesn't mean you can't have the sugary juice or cappuccinos again! It's the **habit** we are aiming to replace—so question yourself whether there might be a better choice, next time you say yes out of habit.

Write a list of your intended habit substitutions and start trying them out one by one. When replacing *the Baddies* for *the Better,* consider the following three points:

1) Remind yourself why you want to change the habit (the benefit).

2) How will you feel by making the substitution?

3) Keep in mind your goal or trigger words from your wellness vision.

Just another tip: if the habit is linked to an existing routine, such as grabbing takeaway every morning on your way to work, look to vary your routine. *No, I'm not suggesting a day off work!*

Weaning (can be risky!)

Varying your habit by cutting down on quantity is a positive step but can be risky, like continuing to feed a drug habit. Take the example of sugar. I know clients who've tried to cut down on the number of teaspoons they have in their coffee and start reducing it by a few

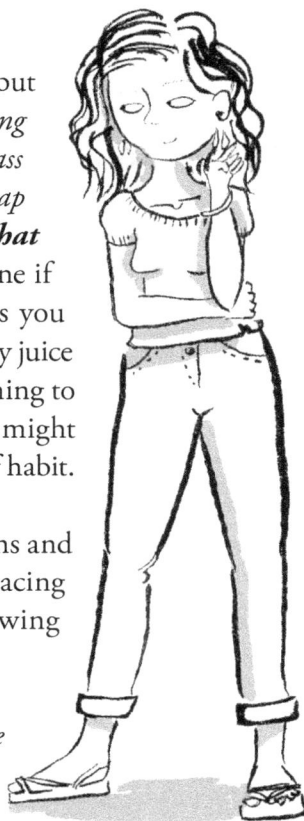

granules every day—it's a slowwwww process. As sugar is so addictive, they are still feeding that habit. Consider the next approach.

Cold turkey

If replacing or weaning off a habit is not working, then you may wish to consider full-blown 'cold turkey'. Be aware that this can be challenging because your brain will be sending you all sorts of messages. If you can find some strong resolve, then do it! I have found that after three consecutive days, it gets easier, so hang in there!

The advantage of the cold turkey approach means that your resolve and determination will get stronger for every day that you stay 'clean'. Saying 'No' will become easy. *'No sugar in my coffee please!'* Be creative to find new solutions. *'I might also replace my coffee with tea during this quit sugar phase because I don't like sugar in my tea anyway'.* One day, someone will make you a coffee with sugar, and you will want to spit it out for tasting sickly sweet. Progress ... bring it on!

3. KNOW YOUR ASSOCIATIONS AND TRIGGERS

Avoid or manage them

We know that repetition is the way to turn those desirable behaviours into habits that stick and here we are cruising along, feeling proud and pumped to be clocking up lots of reps on the repetition path, just like muscle memory. We are blitzing our goals and winning the game of habits by practising our new strategies! Then BANG CRASH!!! What was easy peasy yesterday is suddenly impossible today. *Why? We were going so well ...*

Other influences can weaken our resolve and act to sabotage our admirable efforts. When we are aware of them, we can be better prepared and take action to mitigate them. Determine when your resolve is poor. Troubleshoot and create your own list of solutions. Here are some of the common ones:

Under the influence: It is easy to become careless and have impaired judgement about healthy choices once we are under the influence of alcohol, drugs, tiredness or stress. When we can't eliminate these things from our lives, we must find ways to better manage them.

Alcohol: If you only ever reach for the addictive crackers or overeat when drinking alcohol, then prepare some nutritious yummy snacks in advance and make sure there are no unhealthy temptations in sight.

Tiredness: It's not always possible to eliminate tiredness. Demanding lifestyles can play havoc with our bodies. Have you found yourself eating more sugary things to prop yourself up after a sleepless night? Do what you can to manage this one. Make every endeavour to create good sleep habits and experiment with power naps, meditation and good nutrition. Refresh with pre-made energising snacks or smoothies from your freezer.

Hormones: Our hormones can influence food cravings. Consult a medical professional for specific advice about the best nutrition and exercise that may help.

Stress: When you can't remove the stress, find ways to manage it. Place the super-size chocolate bars out of sight—forget about those brown paper bags in the top cupboard. Exercise is a great stressbuster along with meditation and mindfulness activities too.

The company we keep: We generally find it easier to stick to our health plans if we are in company that shares similar views that match our desired habits. This can be tricky when we don't have a say in who our workmates are. Perhaps you work alongside the 1970s version of Norm from 'Life be in it' ads? Or maybe you are surrounded by temptation at family gatherings? Beware of 'sabotaging' behaviour from others to justify their own choices.

Problem solve your own best strategies ahead of time, and practise saying 'No'. The more you say 'No', the stronger your resolve will be, which will reinforce a positive mindset encouraging you on in your quest for better health. Keep clear of Norm or invite him into your circle—his habits may change for the better too!

4. ASSOCIATIONS

'I have to eat something sweet after dinner'; 'I cannot leave food on my plate'; 'I always have two sugars in my coffee'; 'I always have two slices of toast, not one'; 'I always have popcorn and a choc bomb at the movies'…

In most cases, the beliefs hold no truth when it comes to improving eating habits and they need to be questioned and altered. Do you want it because you need it or want it just because it is what you have always done in the past? Bring more awareness to your actions by pausing to reflect on why you are doing something. Change up your routine. If you always have a cuppa and biscuit after dinner, then organise a walk or other activity in its place. When going to the movies, challenge yourself to bypass the candy bar.

Q&A

Q. How can I become more committed to building new habits?

Find a buddy to be accountable to or enrol your family and friends to join you in a challenge.

Q. I have lots of habits I'd like to change and not sure where to begin …?

Many people get so enthused about change that they overdo it. Don't rush the process! Master one or two simple habits before moving on to the next. This will build confidence and ensure your long-term success.

Q. I have good intentions of creating new healthy habits but keep procrastinating about starting. How can I overcome this?

Adopt the 'two-minute rule' suggested by James Clear in his book *Atomic Habits*. Make the habits as easy as possible to begin by scaling them down into two-minute versions. Establish the practice first and then improve on it. For example, *'Write in my journal each night'* becomes *'Jot down three sentences about my day'*. *'Complete 30 minutes of exercise'* becomes *'Do 12 squats'*. *'Tidy my room'* becomes *'Put five items away'*. Start today!

IN A NUTSHELL:

- **Practise conscious awareness** of your unwanted behaviours and recognise whether they happen from choice or a habit. If conscious, try delay tactics.

- **Assess and write down** some habits that don't align with your goals or vision. Aim to replace, wean or go cold turkey to discard the Baddies. If you are eliminating them, commit to three days in a row to kickstart the process.

- **Create your own list of habit substitutions** for any habits you wish to change.

- **Repeat good behaviours** until they become habits to support your desired goals.

- **Don't try to tackle too many habits at once.** Start small with one or two and practise getting control over your choices. It will help you grow confidence before moving on to some more.

- **Be patient** on the journey of self-awareness, instead of thinking about the end date. If you slip up, don't stress; learn from it and change up routines. Get back on board.

- **Take small steps** to build success. Focus on daily wins of continuous improvement.

'We first make our habits, and then our habits make us.'

– John Dryden

CHAPTER 8

Who Ya Gonna Call?
Your support team

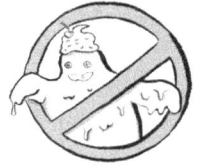

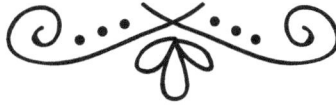

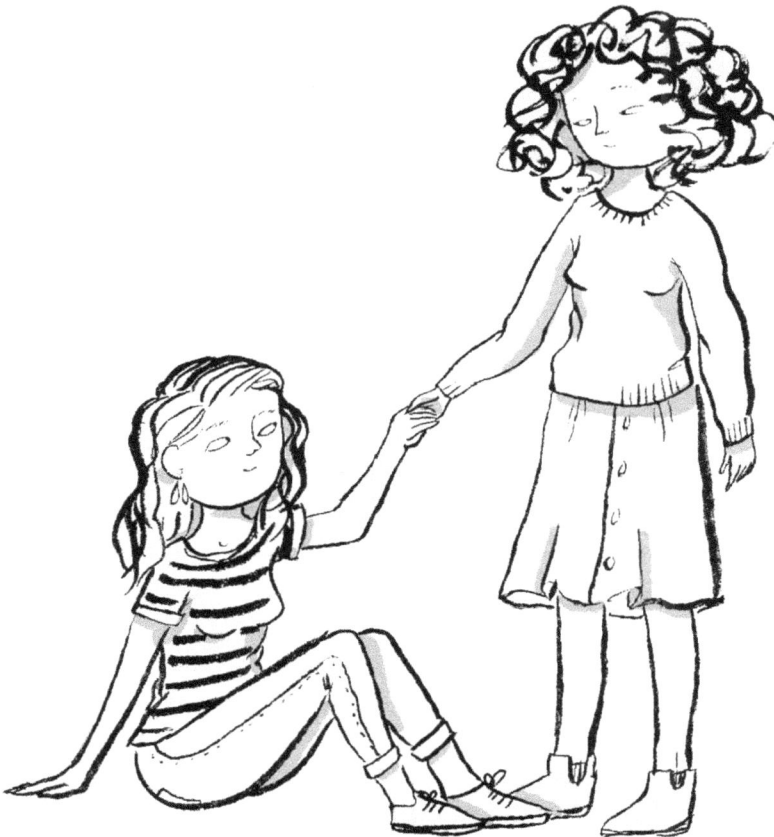

'Ask for help. Not because you are weak. But because you want to remain strong.'

– Les Brown

E ven the most independent of us can benefit from support on our wellness journey. Who knows **what** is around the corner? We can be cruising down Easy Street with a spring in our step and the world at our feet and then ... BANG! We hit a wall! That's when our support team comes in.

Support can come in the form of practical help to learn a new skill or get advice. It may be emotional support—a sympathetic ear, someone to cheer us on or boost morale.

There may be times when we are reluctant to ask for help. It could be shyness or lack of confidence, or we might be downright independent and too proud to ask. Surely, we can benefit from a helping hand, so what other reasons hold us back?

If we speak it out loud and ask for help, we might have to give up excuses and take action or be accountable to someone else. *Damn! Now I'll have everyone bombarding me with questions and checking up on me.*

If we don't ask for help, we can stay in our comfort zone and won't have to do anything! That's the good news. If, however, you are sick and tired of staying in comfort or limbo land and want to improve your health, then asking for support will ensure you carry through with your intentions. It really is your choice.

I've reflected on not taking action sooner to regain my health after having children and struggling with it. *Why* didn't I ask for help earlier?

Pride got in the way and feelings of being incompetent if I couldn't manage to do this on my own. I'd had a successful corporate career and been extremely capable. I had to accept that I was not perfect, nor was I that same person. It was okay to be feeling a little lost in my new role and need strategies to find my way forward.

It seems an obvious thing to just ask for help, but it involves swallowing some pride and coming out of hiding to say: *I'm not coping, I'm serious about change, I need help!*

How do you ask for help?

Others are not mind-readers, nor do they want to hurt your feelings by suggesting help if you are not ready to hear it.

'Whingeing' is *not* asking for help. All those years ago, I probably said things like *'I've got NOTHING to wear—all my clothes are too tight!'* in a frustrated 'under my breath' way to no-one in particular. How could anyone even know what type of help I actually wanted?

We need to be clear about voicing our desire for help in the form that **we** want. To use direct communication: *'I'm unhappy with how I'm feeling. I want to improve my health and need your support by ...'*

Well-meaning friends and partners can intend to be supportive by either telling you what you *should* do (unhelpful unless you've asked for their opinion), or suggest that you don't need to change a thing (only helpful if they understand what YOU want). If you are serious about wanting changes around your health, then take back the reins and enlist the right help.

Choose the best people on your team

Choose your team based on the level of practical and emotional help they can offer. You may not need any immediate help, but it is still wise to have your team considered in advance.

The advantages

- Sharing with others can make the journey fun as you support each other.
- Your support team can help you feel connected to others and make new friends.
- Receiving good support, can in turn, make you a great help to others.
- You can learn from professionals quickly or from those who have tread the same path.
- Others can encourage you when motivation is lacking and allow you to lean on them to get back on track.
- Learning to accept help can give you a sense of freedom—*I don't know it all! I'm human and I'm not perfect! I don't need to have all the answers!*
- Asking for help is another step towards commitment. Announcing it to the world (or just a few) means you are serious. It will also give you accountability.

If you don't have a support structure in place, others may unintentionally sabotage your efforts through not understanding. It could take longer to achieve by trial and error, and it can also be a lonely journey.

Here are some tips for choosing your team and how they can help you.

1. SELECT YOUR SUPPORT TEAM

Who do you want on your team now or in the future? My team includes family, friends, business mentors, fellow members in clubs and groups, work colleagues, my doctor, naturopath, chiropractor, physiotherapist, personal trainer and a range of other allied health professionals.

Write a list of who can offer emotional and practical support. This list is going in your toolbox! Here are some suggestions:

- **Family and friends** can give you that deep personal connection and understanding.
- **Health professionals, coaches and experts** can teach you new skills and fast-track your progress with professional help. They can also provide motivation and emotional support.
- **Work colleagues and neighbours** that you see on a regular basis can offer support and recognition of your efforts.
- **Other acquaintances** can help you with practical assistance such as someone to share lifts to a class or a babysitter to mind the kids.
- **Clubs** provide an opportunity to meet new people and develop networks.
- **Groups** can provide good support from like-minded people that have similar goals to you. It's also an opportunity to help and learn from each other.

2. *YOU* DECIDE HOW THEY CAN HELP

You make the rules!
You call the shots and direct your support people how they can best help you.

- When visiting medical or fitness professionals, don't assume they will know what you want. Be specific in what you want to achieve or how you or are feeling. *'I want to start running and don't know where to start.'*
- If the person does not have good listening skills, then find someone who does—preferably someone who connects with eye contact and is not writing or typing the whole time you are talking. *A friend of mine was mildly overweight and went to a fitness specialist. Before she could explain her reason for the appointment, he started on how he could help her lose weight. That wasn't what she wanted help with—she wanted to build strength in her legs prior to a knee op!*

- Inform your family and friends what you are doing. Request them to give you the help that you ASK for (not what *they* think you need).
- Ask them NOT to police you (unless that's what you want). Suggested conversations include: *'Please don't keep asking me how much weight I've lost—I don't want our whole conversation to be about my diet.'; 'I'm not great with the power of suggestion, so please don't offer me a glass of bubbly with dinner.'; 'If you want your own stash of chocolate, can you keep it secretly stored in a brown paper bag?'; 'Pour yourself a glass of wine, but don't leave the wine bottle on the table.'* Perhaps they will be inspired and join you in some new healthy habits too.
- Find other ways for people to support you. If you are trying to lose weight or eliminating sugar or alcohol, suggest social catchups that don't revolve around food or drink. Ask your friends to get on board with *walk n talk* in place of *coffee and cake.*

3. CALLING IN HELP

So, you know **who** they are and **how** they can help, but is that enough? Try setting up some strategies to ensure that you actually *utilise* their help and they don't just stay as a name in your toolbox.

Prearrange appointments: Pre-planning is my number one strategy. If we wait until we *feel* like it or until we hit a roadblock, we may never move (or start)! Say things like *'Let's walk every Monday at 9 am. Lock it in!'*

Use your diary: Set up regular sessions with friends, personal trainers and others on your team. Consistency is paramount.

Update them: At home, dedicate a regular time to update your family and have discussions about their ongoing support ... *Don't police me!*

Keep the chocolates hidden! Discuss celebratory rewards that involve them.

Turn up—be consistent: Don't cancel arrangements unless it's super urgent or you are ill. If an appointment has to be cancelled, reschedule immediately.

Sending out an SOS: There will be times when pre-planning is not enough and when something hits the fan, reach out to your team for support to share the load, vent or talk it out.

Express gratitude: Keep your support team informed with as much as you are happy for them to know. Be grateful that they are on your team and tell them so!

Pay it forward: Look for opportunities to support others. There is the added advantage of learning that comes from helping others, and we also get to appreciate that we are not alone in our challenges.

Q&A

Q. What if I live alone and don't have friends to support me?
Join social clubs or groups in your area; you may surprise yourself with some new ideas and good company. Social media, Facebook—there are many groups online where you can share your story and get support.

Q. What if I'm trying to lose weight and my partner keeps telling me that I'm fine the way I am? He always wants to order in pizza!
Get a new partner!!! Just kidding. Ask him to support you—the health benefits and weight loss will benefit you both. Respect your partner's needs too and reach a compromise, such as cooking a healthy pizza together—it's great fun. Consider an occasional home delivery.

Q. What if I'm self-motivated and don't think I need anyone to support me?

It's great to have that motivation and confidence. Treat this as insurance that you may never have to use and don't forget your network will work both ways.

IN A NUTSHELL:

- **Make a list** of who your support people are and what they can do for you.

- **Consider how your team can best support you.** Talk to them and give them your 'rules'.

- **Use a diary** and make regular pre-planned appointments. Be consistent.

- **Don't struggle in isolation.** Reach out for help when you need it.

- **Express gratitude for your support team** and look for opportunities to be supportive to others.

CHAPTER 9

Mastering Mindset and Motivation
Generating positivity

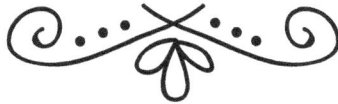

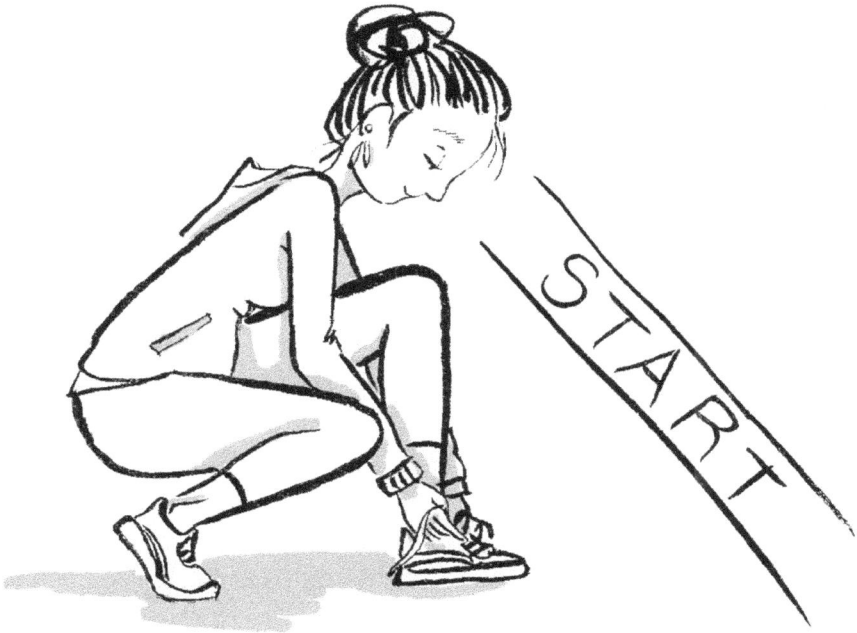

'The secret of getting ahead is getting started.'
– Mark Twain

I love to crank up my 70s and 80s music often! Nothing unusual about that, however sometimes I switch from easy listening to hot disco, when it is actually the LAST thing I *feel* like doing … Why?

It's one of my personal strategies to rev myself up enough to head out the door for the walk I promised myself if I'm feeling like I need an extra push to get my trainers on. By the way, seeing as I didn't get much sleep and I'm not feeling 100 percent, I've also given myself permission to adapt the 30-minute planned walk to just 10 minutes. It's about keeping the commitment going.

Often, movement builds momentum. By the time I've done 10 minutes, I've generated some energy and might decide to go another round or three around the block. OMG that just turned into an hour of Donna Summer and suddenly I'm not so tired after all! How did that even happen?

Sometimes we don't *feel* like doing something, even meeting up with a friend for a walk that was prearranged. Perhaps we are not in the mood and want to cancel. You don't because the thought of your friend waiting expectedly for your arrival is a good reason to show up. You go on to have the walk, unwind, catch up and feel pumped with endorphins. Reflecting back later, you are glad you didn't cancel. It highlights the great benefits of accountability and prearranging strategies, particularly around exercise.

Cultivating a positive mindset and finding strong motivation can help us experience that wonderful energy flowing through our body, compelling us to take action and bring our vision to life. It will also:

- build confidence and self-belief
- influence and improve our relationships
- prepare us for the unexpected before it happens
- address unhelpful filters and internal chatter that is not serving us.

If we don't plan to manage our mindset, we risk losing motivation and may quit when it is not what we really want to do.

Many strategies can help pull us out of a slump and generate positive motivation but first, we will start by delving into your mindset.

PART A: MINDSET

'We cannot solve our problems with the same level of thinking we used when we created them.'
– Albert Einstein

Mindset is your personal collection of thoughts, attitudes, stories and beliefs that shape your behaviours and habits, consciously and subconsciously.

When researching into the fascinating world of mindset, I interviewed my 15-year-old daughter who enlightened me on the topic. In Year 4 at primary school, they learned about the theory of *growth vs. fixed mindset*. My daughter reassured me this was a fairly new concept and would not have been around when I went to school! She was right and I set out to explore.

I discovered the founder of the growth mindset theory, Carol Dweck, Professor of Psychology at Stanford University. In 2006, she published *Mindset: The New Psychology of Success*. The book describes the importance of having the right mindset to maximise our potential and capitalise on our strengths. The main difference between the two mindsets, is that *fixed* beliefs hold little or no room to change, while the *growth* mindset is open to change, and seeks opportunities for improvement or growth.

Professor Dweck's TED talk had me thinking about a word that she focused on when developing a growth mindset—the word 'yet'. For example, *'I'll never get through this book'* changes to *'I haven't been able to get through this book **yet**'.* There is so much power in one word and it opens up a whole new mindset possibility.

I'd been curious about the various mindsets of my clients. When incorporating a fun factor into personal training sessions based on balance skills, their reactions were varied. When giving them a challenging task that they had never tried before, I would get varying responses from: *'You've got to be kidding me, I could never do that'*, *'No way, my balance is useless'*, to *'Bring it on, I'd love to try!'*

I wondered how their response might change if they had greater awareness to cultivate a growth mindset? One that enabled them to reframe their answer to: *'I don't know if I could do it'* or threw in the word *'yet'*.

We are not all drawn to like the same challenges; however, I was interested in knowing why people responded in a certain way and how their mindset was involved. From reviewing Professor Dweck's theory, if they were more inclined to have a growth mindset, but their response came from thoughts of not wanting to look foolish or fear of failing, I could help instil confidence in their abilities. None of their responses are right or wrong. It just demonstrates how different people react and how I could also get a variable response from the same client on a different day. Our internal chatter can be positive on some days (help me stand on that fitball now) to days when a negative mindset has the same client cancelling the gym session.

According to the growth mindset theory, our mindset determines the way we deal with tough situations and setbacks. It also determines our willingness to improve ourselves through our passions and goals.

A predominately fixed mindset means you believe that your abilities, attributes and intelligence are inherently fixed and unchangeable. If you have a predominantly growth mindset, then you see the possibilities of learning and trying things out with a flexible attitude.

I also gained valuable learning from reading books and articles around mindset by Dr Stephanie Burns, an international leader of brain and mind research who has shaped my thoughts on this topic. I first read her book *Great Lies We Live By*, over 25 years ago! I re-read the book when I started out as a personal trainer. Her thoughts on choosing our beliefs and changing our internal dialogue, helped me to understand how important mindset awareness was, particularly when it came to coaching others.

I introduced many of her ideas to my training sessions. I reassured new clients that were just starting out, that they 'did not look silly'— they were just in a learning phase as a 'beginner'. Coaching clients to rephrase their beat-up comments is a great way to increase their confidence. Drawing on the knowledge I've learned from Dr Burns, and from Dweck's growth mindset theory, I've shared below three key areas to help you become more aware of your own mindset to bring possibilities for change.

1. MINDSET AWARENESS

Become aware
Practising personal awareness when faced with decisions, will take you closer to your goal. If you can bring awareness to a fixed mindset, you will have a choice of staying in that mindset or not. Talk back to it! Question yourself!

How to assess?
The stories we tell ourselves, our habits and choices are all good indicators for assessing our mindset. Start by asking questions about the choices you make concerning your health and fitness. Test if what you think or say to yourself is actually true or merely a belief. There's a lot more room for growth with 'beliefs'.

Consider questions such as:

- Are we making that choice through the filters of stories we tell ourselves?
- Does the choice appear automatic through habits that we have done for so long, we believe they are part of who we are?
- Are we making conscious choices to keep comfortable and away from the fear of failure?

How does awareness help?

Becoming aware of your mindset brings a realisation that there is fluidity and choice to reframe your thinking and habitual (auto) response. Try looking at situations through a growth lens, rather than a fixed mindset lens. It will help you to explore more possibility in situations where you have previously been held back from trying something new, due to a self-limiting belief.

Awareness can keep you comfortable in a fixed mindset or ready to explore what a growth mindset could mean to you. For example: *'I can't do push-ups'* or *'I don't like gyms'* to *'I'm not great at push-ups **yet**'* and *'I don't know if I like gyms but am open to finding out'*.

2. CHANGE YOUR INNER DIALOGUE

What you say to yourself will affect what you do. I've encountered clients who say things like *'I could never go to an exercise class. I'm not coordinated enough'*, *'I've never been sporty, I can't run'*, *'I'm not a morning person'*, *'I could never do what you do'*. Perhaps that's true, but at least explore *why* you think that. If you don't try, you will never know. Ask yourself, what would it take to change your beliefs?

The power to choose your beliefs

By adopting this thinking, it will open the door to the possibility for change *if we want it*. We can choose to stay comfortable. In fact, this can be quite appealing, like staying in bed on a cold winter's morning. This can, however, come at a cost of personal disappointment for missing out on a new experience—like telling yourself, *I can't get out of bed before sunrise.* If we have the desire, we can change that internal dialogue and move beyond it.

I considered the language of clients which influenced their behaviours. One of my clients Connie, was not prepared to limit herself through a lack of natural talent and ability. She displayed a generalised growth mindset whilst holding some fixed beliefs about her abilities.

Connie was heading for a milestone birthday—the big 'five-oh'. Her fears revolved around what other people might think and what if she tried something and failed. Those fears had kept her safely sheltered on the couch as she secretly dreamed about one day joining a fun run and even a triathlon event.

She'd been snoozing comfortably through life, a woman in her 40s with unrealised dreams. Her aha moment came with an inspirational story on TV, about someone who had defied all the odds to learn to walk again after an accident. The couch was suddenly too spongey as she battled to sit up and calculate how many months until her birthday. Her meter was about to tick over. She realised time was running out—she must explore those dreams and get off the couch. But how to start? We talked. She told me 'I don't know how to run. I look like a waddling duck!'. She went on to explain that she didn't LOOK like what a runner was meant to look like …, 'Well I'm short, dumpy, my fat wobbles, my boobs bounce, I gasp for breath. I can't breathe properly.'

This mindset of self-doubt and worrying about looking foolish had kept Connie in a state of inaction. The thought of a fun run or triathlon had been filed away in the 'impossible' basket and up until this moment, she had never started to attempt *any* running. She felt disappointed and lacked confidence.

Connie had already begun her journey by having the courage to speak out loud what had been in her head and what was influencing her mindset. Before I could assess if running was a physical possibility, we had to talk further about her mindset.

This highlights the importance of addressing mindset issues that go hand in hand with physical capabilities. Whilst a *growth mindset* got her off the couch, we needed to work on her *fixed mindset* about her actual capabilities.

Changing internal dialogue

Connie's inner dialogue was full of self-criticism, fear and doubt. She had to overcome her inner dialogue that shouted out:

You can't run!
You'll never be able to keep up—you get puffed out running to the letterbox!
You are short and dumpy and don't look like a runner!
You waddle like a duck!

Before any physical training started, we set about changing her beliefs from *'I can't run'* to *'I don't know if I can run, yet'* and *'I want to learn how'*.

We did this by finding out whether her statements were true or merely beliefs. She then had the power to challenge them.

I had heard Dr Stephanie Burns say that your internal dialogue programs your brain towards success or failure. Your brain doesn't care whether you learn

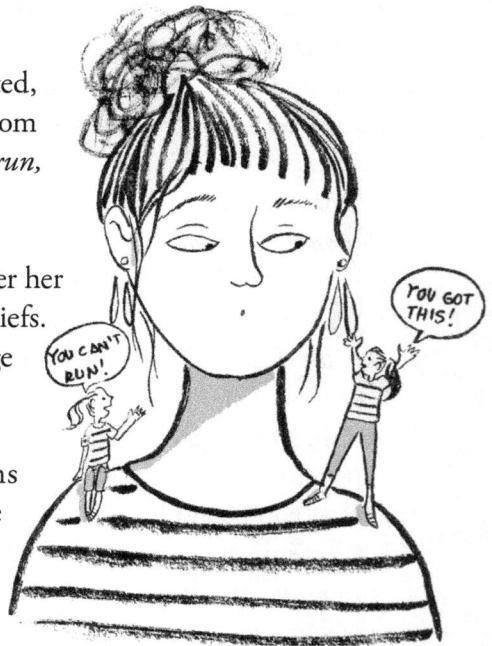

128

how to do something or not. Your brain wants to be right and will direct your behaviour to match your expectations.

'Whether you think you can, or you think you can't, you're probably right.'

– Henry Ford

3. EMBRACE NEW OPPORTUNITIES FOR GROWTH

Learning is an opportunity for growth

When learning a new skill, challenges and failures are part of the learning process. The way you respond to them can be the difference between success and failure. Don't give up because you're not the best at something. Enjoy the learning process with patience and persistence. The *growth mindset* will use challenges as opportunities for growth.

Learning does not mean perfecting it. If we only focus on instantly mastering a new skill whilst still on our L plates, we may give up prematurely through unrealistic expectations. We can worry about looking foolish. Don't compare yourself with others and do the best you can within your own set of capabilities.

Everyone needs to start somewhere

When learning any new skill, whether it's running, squats or push-ups, be prepared to be vulnerable and LOOK like a beginner. I reassure my beginner gym clients with this often. Everyone has to start somewhere, so aim to enjoy the entire process, not just the outcome. Be okay to start with beginner push-ups to the wall, supported squats and so on.

Whilst Connie was successful and confident as a computer analyst, she had to realise that in the area of running, she was a beginner! At this starting out point, Connie had to overcome her fear of looking silly. She did not look like a triathlete—*yet.*

Bite size chunks

This bite size chunk approach is also discussed in goal setting, but I'd like to continue with Connie's story to give you the full picture of how her growth mindset made her goals a reality.

We created a vision that was now becoming a real possibility. The vision brought her fun run and triathlon dream into the realms of possibility, and gave meaning to Connie's reasons for changing her inner dialogue and create new behaviours and habits.

Connie was feeling overwhelmed on how to bring this vision to life. We had to break down some goals around the vision into bite sized chunks, consistently and with support. One step at a time. We needed to change Connie's mindset from overwhelm to *I think this is possible.*

This step by step approach had us doing very short runs on the basketball courts and lots of repetitive learning drills to learn about technique, cadence and breathing. Each week we would add on additional runs to the previous week's attempt. I was so proud of her determination and commitment.

I helped Connie with mindset and other tools like goal setting as well as some basic foundational running skills. As I am no expert in running, I referred her to a specialised running clinic. She had developed confidence and practised saying to herself, '*I can run, I don't look silly. I'm getting better at this. I can do this*'.

I continued to train Connie in the gym to develop overall strength and flexibility and enjoyed hearing of her latest achievements. She'd migrated from the basketball court to football ovals and had now signed up for a charity fun run event.

Connie did get to take part in the fun run. She didn't win a place, but she certainly won her own personal best achievement of participating and didn't *waddle like a duck*. She went on to use these same mindset tips to question her beliefs in other areas. She booked specialist coaches and has now successfully completed in several triathlon events. Her confidence is sky high as she contemplates her next challenge.

SOME FINAL TIPS ON MINDSET

Support your learning

- Don't keep it all in your head. Question yourself, speak it out loud. Call in professional help or a trusted friend to bring about a fresh perspective and to help you challenge your beliefs.
- Be inspired by listening to podcasts or reading motivational books or biographies on everyday people overcoming challenges.
- Cultivate the courage to get off the couch and waddle like a duck! Transport yourself into slightly *uncomfortable*.

Remember, when learning a new skill:

- it's fine to make mistakes
- trust and believe in your abilities and do the best you can
- don't give up—it is not that you can't, you are not able to—**yet**
- focus on progression with the task becoming easier each time.

Reframe your dialogue

Next time you have an issue around mindset, change your inner dialogue and reframe that story:

'I'm not a morning person' to *'I don't know if I'm a morning person'*.

'I could never get up before sunrise' to *'Others can do it, why don't I at least try.'*

'I can't sit still to meditate' to *'I want to find out if I can become someone that enjoys daily meditation'*.

Whether it's a physical skill or a belief around being able to meditate, how will you know what's possible, if you don't try? Become aware of your mindset and explore the possibilities of changing it.

Quieten your mind

Try meditation and give your brain a break from all the mental chatter going on. You will feel refreshed and better able to recognise when it's all just in your head.

Mantra

Remind your brain and reinforce your decisions—create your own mantra to help you with this. A mantra may also be a song to reinforce positive feelings.

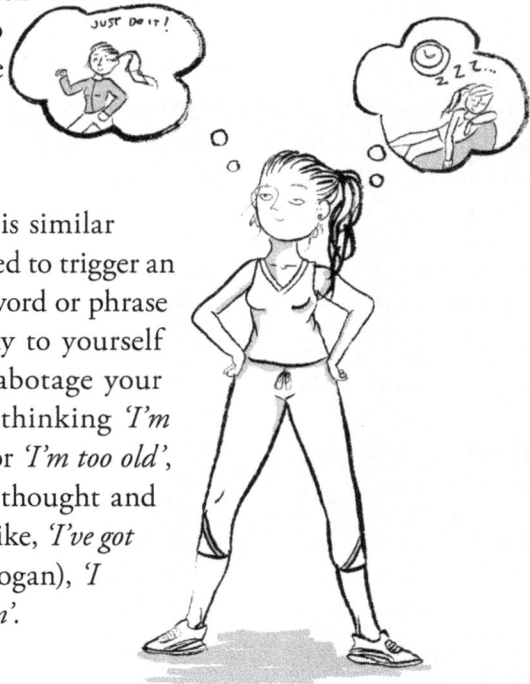

Catchphrase

A personal catchphrase is similar to a mantra. It can be used to trigger an association. It can be a word or phrase that you consciously say to yourself if your mind tries to sabotage your intentions. If you start thinking *'I'm too tired'*, *'I'm too busy'* or *'I'm too old'*, recognise that negative thought and counter it with a phrase like, *'I've got this'*, *'Just Do It'* (Nike slogan), *'I can. I will'* or *'Bring it on'*.

Modify your plans if you are tired but don't give up. Do the 10-minute walk instead of the planned 30. *Just do it*. Write your catchphrase or trigger words on a sticky note and pop it on your water bottle or phone as a reminder.

PART B: MOTIVATION

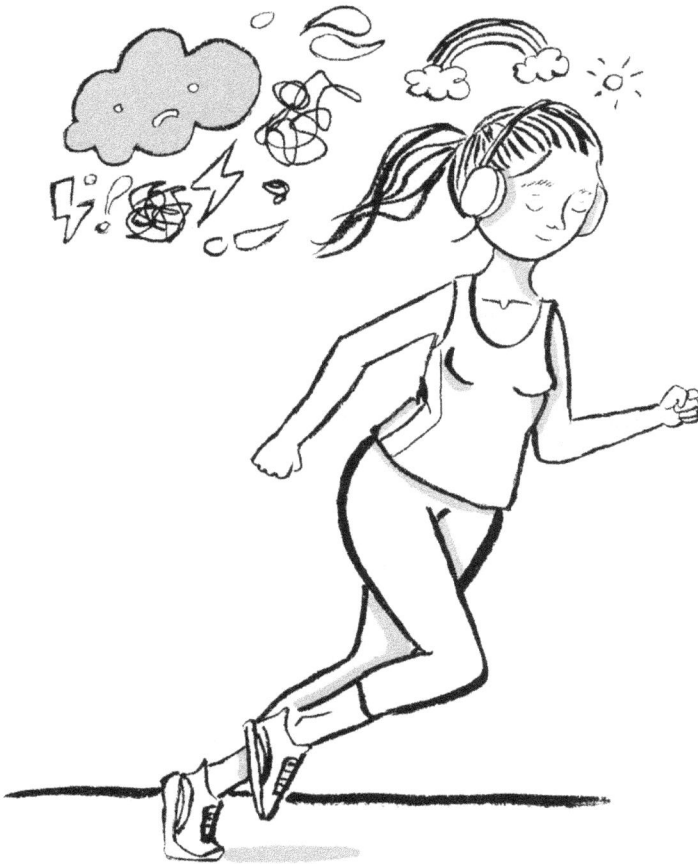

'You're only one workout away from a good mood.

– Anonymous

Staying motivated helps keep you positive and doing your best. We will lose motivation sometimes due to tiredness, imbalance of hormones or feeling stressed. This is life. We can be up and excited mostly, but realistically, there will be down days too.

Name it

Deal with *why* we feel unmotivated. Is it a physiological response or is it stemming from emotions linked to our mindset or mood? Find out why. Talking it out will be helpful.

If we put a name to it, we can accept and validate those feelings as real and choose how to move forward without blame or excuses. The low will be temporary, and you can choose to adapt the plans you made yesterday by trying out the strategies I've listed below.

Sharing our thoughts with a helpful friend or social group can elevate our mood. Sometimes there can be underlying reasons for feeling down that will require expert medical or psychological help. If you feel this is the case, seek assistance from a medical professional.

1. EVERYDAY REINFORCEMENT

Look at your wellness vision regularly
Remind yourself of all the advantages of making changes in line with your wellness vision. Don't keep your vision hidden away. Keep reinforcing the reasons and benefits to your brain.

2. SOCIALISE TO KEEP MOTIVATION HIGH

Stay connected

Nourish good friendships and stay in touch with people that inspire and support you. Mix with like-minded people or those who are on a similar path to you.

Group training kept my motivation high week after week until it became my new best habit and something that I just did.

3. CREATE YOUR TOOLBOX OF STRATEGIES

Pre-planning—baby come back!

Plan your strategies in advance when you *are* feeling good. You will be more receptive to techniques that you know will work for you.

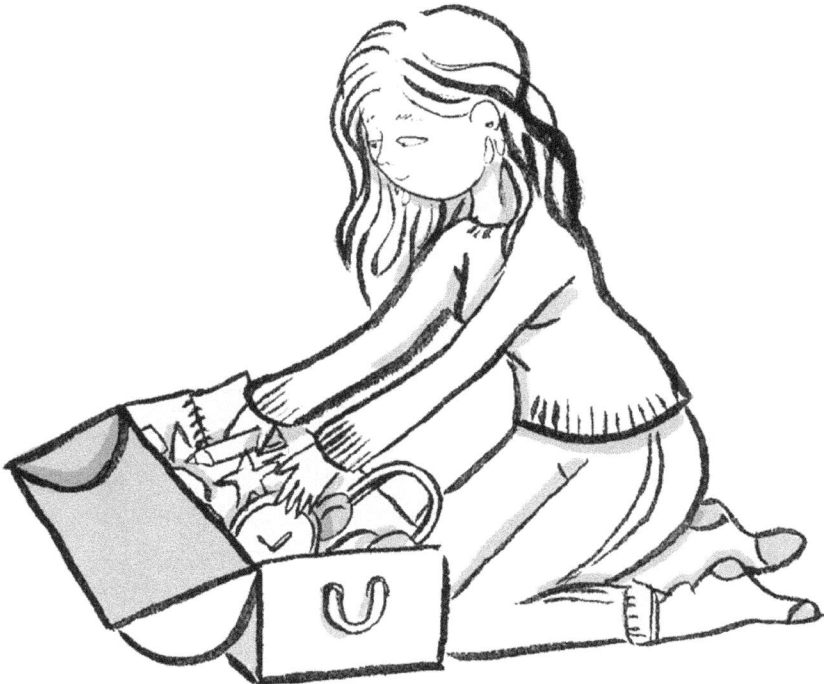

Create your own Bring it Back Toolbox. Write down all the strategies that you know will lift your spirits and reclaim motivation.

For example: *'**If I don't feel like** going for my daily 30-minute power walk, **then I will** get dressed in my workout gear, put on my favourite music and go anyway, even for 10 minutes.'*

What works for one person won't necessarily be effective for another. Here are some of my tips below—but be your own expert.

TIPS to boost your motivation:

Pre-planning: I love having a personal trainer. People say, *'Why are you having PT when you know what to do?'* I am human and open to getting off track and tired as well. I also know that I'll love it when I'm there, or I will love the way I feel *after* the session. It's unrealistic to believe we can love every minute of doing something whilst in the midst of it but loving how it makes you feel, makes it all worthwhile. Pre-planning and pre-paying for my personal training sessions ensures I get to feel this way every week (thanks Russ).

Music: Playing a song that can lift your mood is a winner. I think I learned this strategy from my mum actually …

Many years ago, my mum was on an all-day shopping expedition in Melbourne City. It was summer, and she was feeling hot and bothered as she wrestled with shopping bags, sore feet and blisters. It was a slow, tiring struggle. Oh yes, and she was walking uphill too (at the top end of Bourke Street). Suddenly, without consciously realising what was happening, she picked up the pace and started striding it out with new invigoration. Why? Her body and brain responded to the jolly, upbeat dance music coming from a store.

She could hardly believe how energised she felt as her feet took on a life of their own, now striding it out to the beat of the music. She actually backtracked and went into the store and bought the album. Way to go Mum!

Tricking your brain ... manufacture motivation for a reward: I recall a situation many years ago when I was working at a law firm. I was lacking motivation, feeling swamped and procrastinating by shuffling and triple handling the papers on my desk ...

It was early Friday morning before the long weekend, and I was inwardly complaining about all the work I would need to do over the long weekend to get my desk cleared. By mid-morning, following a phone call, I suddenly had stacks of motivation. What changed? I received a last-minute surprise invitation to go to Singapore for the long weekend. You wouldn't believe how fiercely focused I became, clearing my 'In Tray', my desk—in fact, my whole office! I managed to achieve so much in the rest of the day so that I could grab this amazing opportunity and rock up to work on Tuesday to a clear, organised desk. I did it!

I often refer back and draw on that experience to know that I CAN generate motivation it if I really want to. *Singapore* is now an associative buzz word for me that I sometimes use to get myself moving!

Perhaps you've had an experience when you've manufactured motivation when you thought it was lost. Here's another example that you might relate to:

You don't feel motivated to do the housework and can't be bothered cleaning up the cluttered lounge room ... you don't feel like it, you're too tired, yet you hate looking at all the mess. You envisage it taking you hours, so instead, talk yourself into staying on the lounge. PING! Suddenly you get a text message to say that your friends will be popping in to visit in 20 minutes ... Skates are on, and you quickly blitz the clean-up in less than 20 minutes and have also generated bucket loads of energy. Sound familiar?

I often use a timer to motivate myself to achieve a task in a certain amount of time. Alternatively, an additional incentive can help to keep motivation high. It could be along the lines of: *'If I can meet my targets of exercise this week, I'm booking a massage'*.

Be inspired by other people: Other people can be a great source of inspiration to motivate us. It can help to reach out to our support team or read or listen to stories about people that motivate us.

Clothing: Have you ever noticed how wearing certain clothes can lift your mood? It can be linked to the physical item—a look, feel, fit or colour, or it may be associated with a memory of when we have worn it previously in a happy situation. If you are feeling a little low on motivation, smarten up. Get out of the PJs or sloppy lounge pants and LOOK how you want to feel!

Colour: Our choice of coloured clothing can influence our moods. Rather than wearing a colour that matches a current low mood, choose up, to one that will inspire you. There's a whole psychology around colours.

Colour therapists believe that colour can harmonise and rebalance you if treated with the right colours, and there is some evidence that colour affects our moods and general wellbeing. In 1958, US Scientist Robert Gerard conducted studies to show that colour could affect appetite, blood pressure and aggression.

Marketing gurus are expert at using this info to their advantage by using colours to evoke a certain mood, for example, within restaurants to motivate us to eat more food! Regardless of the science, I know that if I need to re-energise or liven up, I will discard the washed-out beige which on another day may look sophisticated, and choose the red or pink to help me feel energised. Try it for yourself to see which colours evoke certain responses in your mood and motivation.

Smell: Some smells act as an association. If you can know what smells motivate or energise you, then add this to your toolbox. I use an electric diffuser. In fact, I have several around the house and use essential oils. If I need motivation, I swap the relaxation blend to an uplifting blend of citrus oils.

Learning inspiration: Use your growth mindset to keep learning and researching. Read biographies, health and motivational books. Even if you know the content, they are good to read as a refresher or to further reinforce to your brain.

Meditation: Meditation will refresh our mind, make us calmer and receptive to new ideas. It can help put things in perspective.

Action: Action builds momentum. Start with small steps and you will often find this builds momentum.

Some of the tips mentioned in mindset above will also assist you with motivation, such as mantras and catchphrases.

Q&A

Q. What if I'm finding it hard to stay motivated to exercise even though I want to?

Check in again on your *why* reasons. Are they powerful and exciting enough to motivate you? Alternatively, visualise how you will feel at the end of the day when looking back, if you do (or don't) exercise!

Q. I often start off well with a new exercise routine but after a few weeks, if I don't see physical results, I give up. How can this time be different?

Perhaps you are too focused on the end result of physical change. Celebrate other outcomes or benefits you've achieved, such as sticking to a regular exercise routine or improvements in areas such as mood or sleep. Has it become easier to exercise? Engaging a fitness professional can bring a new perspective and ensure you are not being too hard on yourself or unrealistic in what is achievable. It can also add variety to ensure you are not stale or bored with your workouts.

Q. What if I need a little extra motivation and my current strategies are not working?
Keep exploring new strategies to add to your toolbox. There are many fun apps to try such as ThinkUp which includes suggestions for positive affirmations that you record in your own voice, and it also adds in background music.

IN A NUTSHELL:

Cultivating a **positive mindset and strong motivation** can help us to persist with achieving our goals and bring our vision to life.

MINDSET

- **Develop awareness** of your mindset and realise there is fluidity and choice to reframe your thinking and response.

- **Cultivate a growth mindset** to keep learning and exploring.

- **Question your beliefs** and see if they are true.

- **Change your inner dialogue** to one that serves and motivates you.

- **Embrace new opportunities** and be okay looking like a beginner. Start using the word 'yet'.

- **Quieten your mind with meditation** to give your brain a break from mental chatter.

- **Create a mantra** or catchphrase to reinforce positive feelings.

MOTIVATION

- **Ask yourself why you feel unmotivated**. Give it a name and accept those feelings with self-compassion. Share it with a friend or support person.

- **Keep reminding yourself why** you want to improve your health and happiness and reinforce that by keeping your vision clearly in mind.

- **Associate with positive people** that nourish, support and inspire you.

- **Create a toolbox** of your own strategies that will help you in those times when you lose motivation. When you are high on motivation, pre-book catchups and exercise sessions, prepare music playlists, and experiment with your own strategies, such as colour and feel-good clothing.

CHAPTER 10

The Magic of Time Out
Find your inner calm

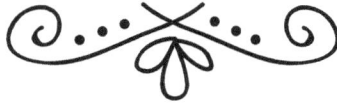

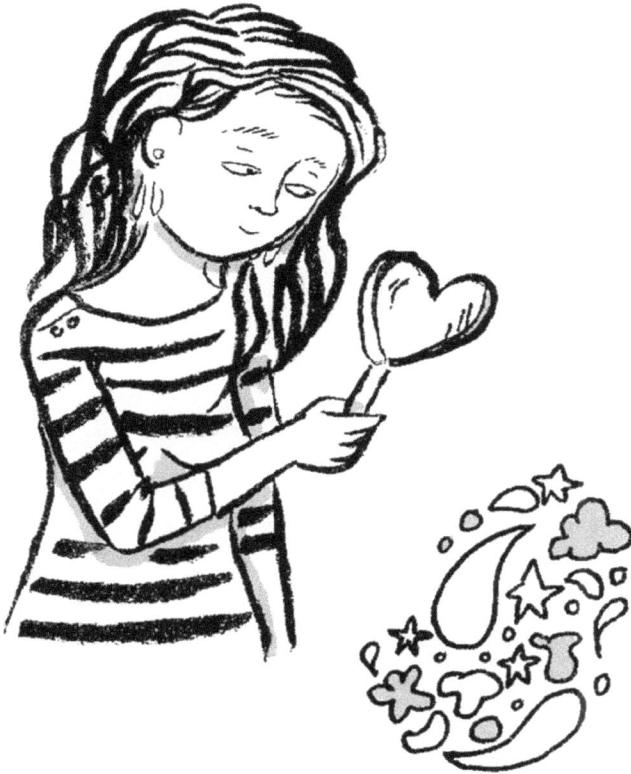

'Your visions will become clear only when you can look into your own heart. Who looks outside, dreams; who looks inside, awakes.'

– Carl Jung

I once heard that substituting **one** word in my daily life could change my outlook on life. It has. Truly. I will share it with you later in this chapter.

Wellness means feeling good about ourselves, physically and mentally—it is influenced by our state of mind and connecting within at a deep level. We know that exercise and good nutrition are key elements of good health and vitality, but proper rest and relaxation are also vital to allow the body to repair and rejuvenate. The mind also needs rest and *time out* from the millions of bits of information we get flooded with every day, as well as the internal chitchat going on in our mind invading our thoughts and clarity.

Stress is a natural fact of life that we all experience to some degree, every day. Stress is not necessarily the villain it is made out to be. In fact, the brain needs a certain level of stimulation, even tension, to function normally. A dull, uneventful daily routine brings along boredom, depression and even disease. But what about stress overload, when we are subjected to *too* much, *too* often and for *too* long? If we neglect our mental wellbeing, our mind and bodies can suffer, leading to ill health.

It is imperative to manage the way we cope with an overload of stress. If we cannot change the events causing it, we need to be well equipped with good coping skills. Physical activity has enormous stress-busting benefits, by reducing levels of the body's stress hormones, such as adrenaline and cortisol, and producing the brain's feel-good neurotransmitters, called endorphins.

Deep breathing and meditation can also cause the body to produce endorphins and are great strategies to help us relax, calm the mind and find clarity to view our lives in a fresh way. Often, just having time out from a stressful situation, can bring on a change of mindset and allow us to find a new solution.

This chapter will look at consciously connecting to the breath as a key strategy to deal with the daily stress of our busy, demanding lifestyles. We will explore meditation, mindfulness and cultivating a gratitude mindset. These practices bring conscious awareness to our thoughts and feelings, restoring calmness, joy and happiness into our lives.

Let's explore four strategies you can incorporate into your everyday life.

1. CONSCIOUS BREATHING

'Feelings come and go like clouds in a windy sky. Conscious breathing is my anchor.'
– Thich Nhat Hanh

Conscious breathing can be grounding, like our own anchor to restore awareness and focus, as Thich Nhat Hanh shares in his quote. As most of our breathing is regulated automatically, conscious breathing can completely shift our perception and enhance specific states of mind and emotions.

During times of stress and inactivity, we often unconsciously shallow breathe, employing only the intercostal muscles to expand the upper chest. In a wellness workshop I attended in Perth many years ago, Dr Carlo Mandofia, MD said, *'We forget about the diaphragm that would act like a pump, filling the lower part of the lungs, but also compressing the liver, spleen, and the intestines—activating the inner rivers, the lymphatic vessels of the abdomen and the large veins returning to the heart.'*

He explained, *'Our lungs always contain a certain amount of air, even when we try our best to thoroughly empty them—it's like water in the oceanic inlets. When we inhale, a tidal wave of fresh air enters our lungs "inlets", mixes with the already existing air and enriches it with oxygen and ionised energy. When we exhale, the tide recedes and carries away the waste, the carbon dioxide.'*

Through **conscious deep breathing**, we will flush our 'inner sea' and improve our vitality. We will fight anxiety, induce a deeper sleep, handle anger or other emotions, meet our inner self, harmonise our body and balance our life. It will also help us relax tension in the muscles, joints and ligaments assisting with mobility and posture.

There are many conscious breathing techniques. The one I share with clients is called 'belly breathing', also known as 'diaphragmatic breathing' or 'abdominal breathing'.

The diaphragm is a large, dome-shaped muscle located at the base of the lungs. Your abdominal muscles help move the diaphragm and give you more power to empty your lungs. Whether you need to calm your nervous system, relax the body, re-energise or tune in to a meditative state, give this breathing technique a try. Practise it for a few minutes every day.

Your guide to belly breathing

When you first learn this breathing technique, practise it either lying down on your back (Version 1), or face down (Version 2) known as crocodile breathing. As it becomes more familiar, it can be done whilst sitting or standing.

Version 1 (belly breathing):

1. Lie on your back in a comfortable position.

2. Put one hand on your belly just below your ribs and place the other hand on your upper chest.

3. Take a deep breath in through your nose and let your belly push your hand out (so it feels like an inflating balloon). Your chest should remain as still as possible.

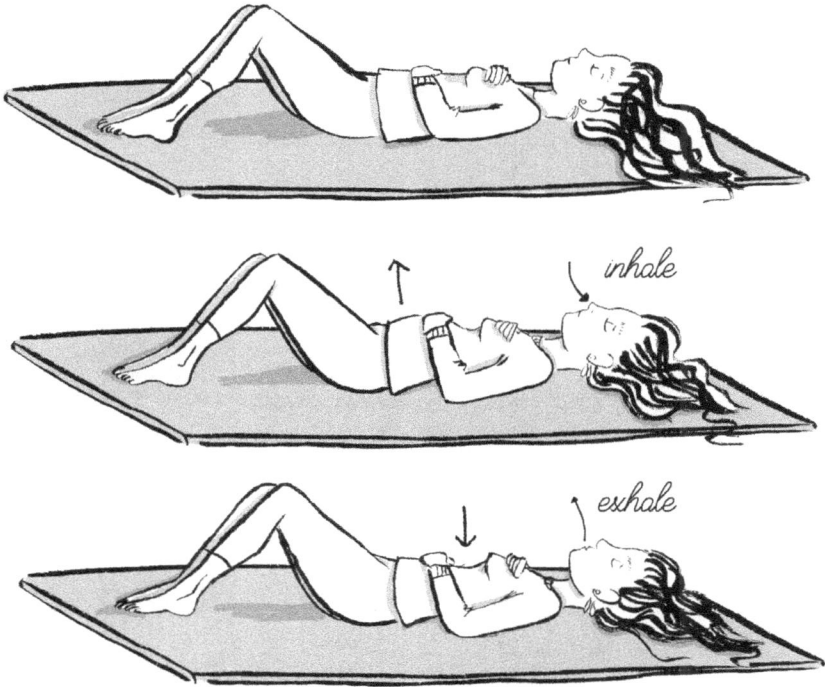

4. As you breathe out through your mouth, draw your belly inward.

5. Allow a natural pause before continuing with the next inhalation.

Version 2 (crocodile breathing):

1. Lay in a prone position (face down) on a firm surface or mat.

2. Rest your forehead on your hands.

3. Take a deep breath in through your nose and let your belly push against the mat.

4. As you breathe out through your mouth, draw your belly inward.

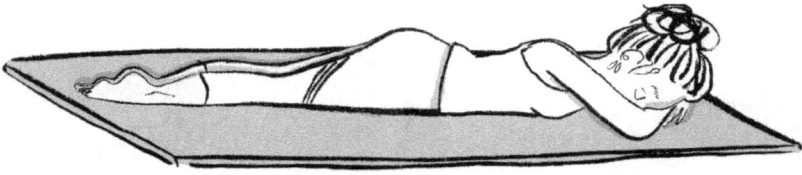

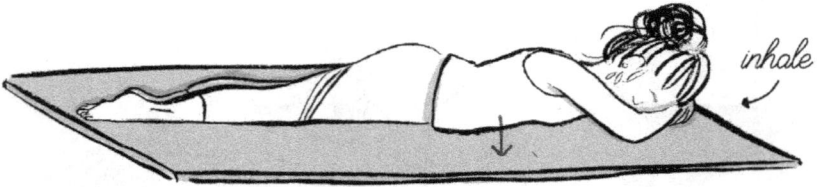

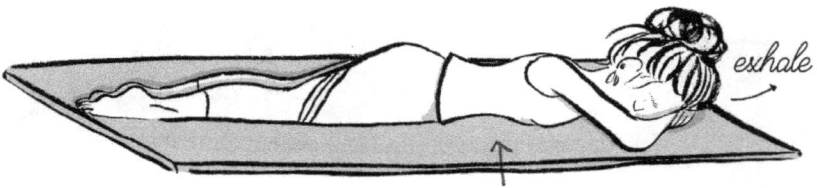

5. Allow a natural pause before continuing with the next inhalation.

TIPS:

- Imagine the breath inhaling vital energy and bathing your brain and every cell of your body with energy and vitality. Use the exhalation as a cleansing way of detoxifying the body.

- The slight pause between the inhalation and exhalation will allow the intercostal muscles, the diaphragm and the abdominal wall to relax for a few seconds. If you find yourself gasping for the next inhalation, then you've paused for too long!

148

2. MINDFULNESS

'The best way to capture moments is to pay
attention. This is how we cultivate mindfulness.'
– Jon Kabat-Zinn

Smell the roses

Mindfulness is a state of being present to the here and now. It could be
when you are pruning roses, enjoying the sensations as you are doing
so with full care and attention—admiring the beautiful velvet-like
petals and smelling the perfume. It is the opposite of doing something
on autopilot, such as cutting back the roses in a hurried fashion whilst
planning your holiday to Bali by speakerphone to the travel agent.
Damn ... those wretched thorns!

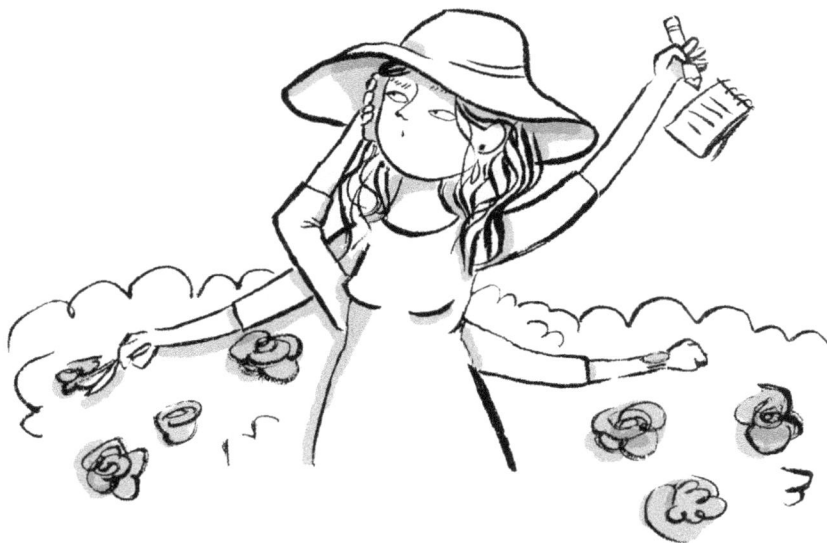

Mindfulness is a skill that takes time to develop. It doesn't have to
be a relaxing experience, although you may feel relaxed when you are
purely focused on the task at hand.

Think of a recent face-to-face conversation you had with someone. Were you present and really listening or were you just hearing part of what they said whilst thinking of other things? Or even cutting their story short so you could interject with your own story? We can all be guilty of this! Practise more mindful listening and notice how your relationships flourish.

Time out

I find that learning a new skill or doing something that involves a high level of concentration can be a great way to experience mindfulness.

Having some mindful 'time out' from any worries can give us a fresh perspective and a drop in overall stress levels.

'Wherever you are, be all there.'

– Jim Elliot

Here are some ideas to incorporate more mindfulness that with regular practice, you can establish new habits around.

- Choose one of your usual everyday activities or tasks and do so with mindfulness. For example, when eating food pay attention to the colours, flavours, textures and taste and savour the experience.

- Enjoy a relaxing walk outdoors, even for a few minutes. Soak up the sights with an appreciation for the beautiful colours of nature. Breathe deeply, take pleasure in the smells and sounds, adopt a sense of curiosity and gratitude to be able to experience the wonder of nature.

- Practise mindful conversation with someone you care about and allow them the luxury of time to express themselves fully.

- Engage in a creative activity such as drawing, mosaics, photography, cooking, gardening, sewing, building, writing, playing a musical instrument or singing.

- Try a few rounds of a mindful breathing by purely focusing on the sensation of your breath.

3. MEDITATION

'Meditation is not a way of making your mind quiet. It's a way of entering into the quiet that's already there—buried under the 50,000 thoughts the average person thinks every day.'

– Deepak Chopra

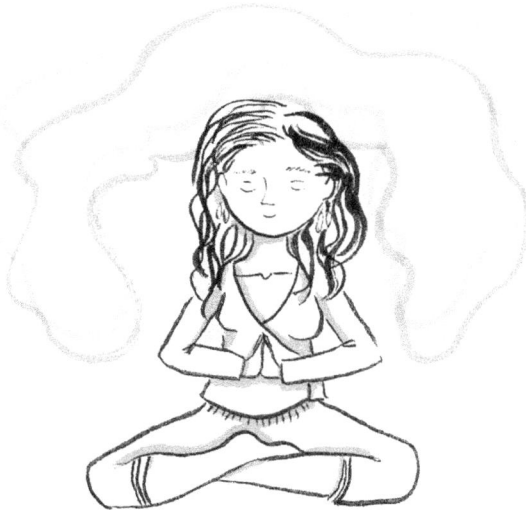

Meditation does not have to mean sitting cross-legged on the floor chanting a vibrational version of '*Ommmm ...*'. There are many styles, and some are even practised during walking or martial arts. It may be

151

done in silence, in nature or to music. It may be a guided relaxation meditation or one focused on the breath. It can be practised at any time of the day for however long you want. It does not have to incorporate any religious component (although it might), and you do not have to be a certain type of person to meditate. Forget structure and rules— it is for everyone!

I had practised some form of meditation before I had a name to label it with, however my first 'formal' introduction to it was back in the 1990s.

At that time, I was working for a city law firm. I worked long hours and always felt in a rush trying to cram in as much as I could. My good friends Richard and Geoff invited me to join them after work for an event. The details were sketchy, but they reassured me it wasn't a network-marketing meeting. Phew!

I'd had a busy day and was dog tired, stressed and really would have preferred to have gone home, vegged on the couch with a glass of wine and some takeaway. I stuck to my commitment but hoped I could go for just a short time and make my escape to get home for an early night.

I raced to meet them straight from the office, having changed clothing from corporate to comfy. I discovered that it was a meditation session being held at a Tibetan Buddhist Centre. That was a first for me and I didn't think it would be 'my thing'. I was a little apprehensive and felt like an imposter, ignorant of rituals and rules.

I was welcomed and made to feel calm and at ease. I was even offered a chair but didn't want to be the odd one out so joined the others on a cushion on the floor. We did various styles of breathing techniques, including alternate nostril breathing and relaxing body scans. I realised how busy my mind was as it dipped in and out of the breathwork to contemplate what I would eat for dinner and my 'to do' list. At those very moments, the meditation master said it was normal to find our mind drifting ...

In his deep reassuring voice, he calmly said not to resist it, but just notice it and gently allow the current of the river flowing past, to carry those thoughts away and bring awareness back to the breath. There was so much freedom in those words, in a world bombarded with rules. I tossed the dinner menu and 'to do' list into the river and felt a deep sense of calm wash over me.

Wow! What an incredible experience this was. Did I feel calm? Yes, but the amazing thing was that the tiredness had totally disappeared and rather than wanting to race home early, I left the class with a huge burst of energy. I felt like I had springs in my shoes and wanted to run and jump about and exclaim how fantastic I felt. I think I DID actually, then went and had coffee and definitely booked in for the next week, month, year or as long as they would let me in! I was hooked! After experiencing many health benefits, I continued to go every week until the centre relocated to the Perth Hills. I'll always be grateful for that beautiful introduction I had to the practice.

Nowadays, I enjoy a few minutes of quiet meditation most mornings, even sometimes staying in bed, whilst listening to a gentle guided morning version and setting an intention for the day ahead. It can also be a great practice to do in the evenings and can help to promote restful sleep.

In my experience, meditation is a chance to experience a taste of timelessness—a time out from the rat race—a time of oneness that calms down, re-centres and yields clarity of mind, peace of heart and equanimity. It is a simple but powerful tool, to give us awareness and clarity, renewed energy and so much more. If you are starting out to try meditation, here are a few more pointers to help you:

- Like many things, meditation is a skill to learn and practise. I won't say *'Practice makes perfect'* because it's not about being perfect. It does not have to involve hours of time. As you become more skilled in meditation and quietening your mind, you will learn to switch to meditation mode quite quickly and can experience great benefits in even a few minutes.

- You don't need to go to a class to learn, although it can be beneficial to learn from an expert. Groups and classes will give you accountability and support. Other options include online programs, podcasts and apps. If you are learning from an app, start with a guided meditation where you are taken through a relaxation exercise for your whole body. I have an assortment of apps on my phone and particularly enjoy the meditations and teachings of Deepak Chopra.

- Develop a new habit for meditation by doing a 21-day challenge or start small with just two minutes of meditation per day and increase over time as that habit becomes part of your everyday life.

- Create a personal sanctuary, such as a small nook or area within your house or garden to practise your meditation. You might want to include a cosy blanket, some cushions and essential oils or balms to have on hand.

4. GRATITUDE

I want to share one particular mindset that has helped me to lower stress and experience more joy: an attitude of gratitude.

Your choice

I promised to share that *one* word that has changed my way of thinking on a daily basis. Okay, I've saved this for the end of the chapter, in the same way that Jack Palance kept us waiting in the *City Slickers* movie, to find out what Curley's '*ONE thing*' was as being the secret to life! When you first hear this 'one word', you may think it unremarkable. Please think about it later though and try it out for yourself. I promise you it works. The implications are powerful and have certainly affected my gratitude mindset.

Substitute *'HAVE to'* with *'GET to'*. So, what does this mean? When you find yourself saying 'I HAVE to …', pause and mentally reframe this in your mind to 'I GET to …'. This has the power to change your mindset about your freedom of choice.

I first heard about this phrase substitution many years ago from Andrew Fuller, a clinical psychologist, author and speaker at a seminar I attended on raising children. I have since heard others mention it, but I'm not sure who to attribute original credit to—but THANK YOU.

Try it out for yourself. *'I HAVE to go to the gym today coz I said I would. Grrr, why did I say I'd go? I don't even feel like it now, it feels like a burden.'* Reframe: *'I GET to go to the gym today coz I said I would but hey, I'm so lucky that I have a healthy body, a car to drive me there and for some people, this is not even possible.'*

'I HAVE to go and pick up my kids from school—why can't they walk like I did as a kid?' Pause, reframe … *'I GET to go and pick up my kids from school. I'm so lucky that I even HAVE kids to pick up from school. Before I know it, they will have left home and I'll be wishing I had that time over again'.*

Imagine there are many people in the world that would gladly trade places with you.

Rephrasing is a way for you to change your whole perspective and inner dialogue around a situation in a positive way.

Sometimes we feel like we have no choice about doing something and can feel really bound to do it. Is someone holding a ransom to you or physically dragging you to do it? Probably not. I guess it's finding *acceptance* of the situation (that you may not be able to change) and trying to create a new possibility around the way you view it, or some crazy advantage. Play with it in your head. It can be creative, just have fun with it. Why? It will transform your mindset from feeling forced and frustrated to an alternative way of thinking that allows for freedom and empowerment as your inner voice calmly tells you ... 'it's your choice.'

Expressing gratitude

That whole 'get to' has really stirred up my sense of gratitude. In positive psychology research, gratitude is associated with greater happiness and wellbeing.

Have you heard of gratitude journals? Gratitude journaling is a way to reflect on things (typically three) that happened in your day that you are grateful for. It doesn't have to be a written journal. Some people use apps, draw or take photos. It's a beautiful way of consciously incorporating more appreciation and gratitude into your life.

We can also reflect on our day and express gratitude verbally. I introduced this to our family as a simple dinner table ritual. We go around the table and share three things that we are grateful for that happened in our day. For example: *I am grateful that our rubbish bin got emptied following our seafood barbeque on the weekend. I'm grateful for the fresh juicy cherry tomato that I grew. I'm grateful that I got to sit in the beautiful sunshine today in my lunch break. I'm extremely grateful for hot running water and toilets that flush!*

For more information on gratitude and positive psychology, take a look at www.positivepsychology.com for a range of inspiring articles and resources.

Q&A

Q. Can conscious breathing help me feel calmer?

Yes. When you are concentrating on your breathing, you are in the present moment. It also calms the nervous system and helps you feel relaxed.

Q. I've tried meditation, but it's not for me. How can I mentally switch off?

Immerse yourself into mindfulness activities—relaxing or not. Even washing the dishes can be meditative! Listening to a podcast is another option. Take one out for a walk!

Q. When I get busy, I sometimes feel guilty if I take time out for myself to relax.

Treat self-care as a priority and factor it into your diary, even if it's only for a 10-minute burst to lose yourself in a good book or laze in a hammock. Incorporate a new calming routine for yourself before bedtime. Experiment with getting up earlier in the morning for gentle stretching, meditation or a podcast.

IN A NUTSHELL:

The mind and body need rest and time out from our busy lives and high levels of stress. Try these techniques to restore balance and bring more joy and vitality into your life.

- **Breathing**: Practise deep conscious breathing. Imagine the breath inhaling vital energy and bathing your brain and every cell of your body with energy and vitality. Use the exhalation as a cleansing way of detoxifying the body.

- **Mindfulness**: Incorporate more mindfulness into everyday activities. Practise mindful conversation, engage in creative activities.

- **Meditation**: Start small, even committing to two minutes every day and increase over time. Enjoy a time of oneness that calms down, re-centres and yields clarity of mind, peace of heart and equanimity.

- **Gratitude**: Next time you feel annoyed and compelled to do something ... pause. Reframe and substitute *'have to'* with *'get to'*. Consciously incorporate more gratitude into your daily life.

CHAPTER 11

Obstacles and Opportunities
Do what you CAN!

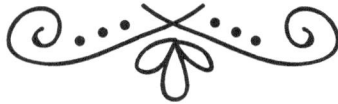

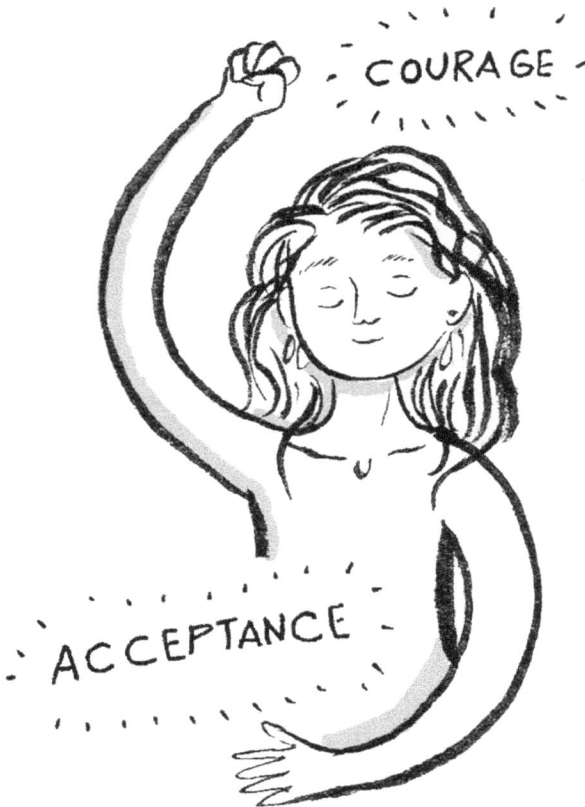

'May I find the serenity to accept the things I cannot change, courage to change the things I can, and have wisdom to know the difference.'
– adapted from the Serenity Prayer

'I can't move! I've got a bad back, walking is impossible!' Is there anything stopping you from starting an exercise program or becoming more physically active when you want to? It can be disappointing when you *want* to be more physically fit but can't. Whether your limitations are permanent or temporary, physical or mental, the focus needs to be on what you **CAN do**—not CAN'T!

Choosing to *accept* what we cannot change helps us to recognise new opportunities, even reap unexpected benefits. It can also make us tougher and more resilient. In difficult times, we don't always find those silver linings immediately. We don't choose to be in situations which turn our worlds upside down. When we are prevented from exercising or eating nutritious meals due to an injury, illness or other obstacle, we do have a *choice* how we view it.

If we fight against it, wishfully thinking 'if only', through the lens of a fixed mindset, rather than accepting it and exploring new possibilities (growth mindset), we can often feed negativity and feel sorry for ourselves. It can become easy to be self-centred and wallow in self-pity.

I know that I have indulged in self-pity after experiencing a setback— after breaking my ankle and not being able to drive. It seems so insignificant now. Feeling sorry for ourselves can be a common response but perhaps it is just part of the process before finding acceptance. What matters is how *long* we stay in that mindset before moving on in whatever way we can.

Dealing with it

It is up to YOU how long it takes to change your mindset. If it is difficult to see beyond today's catastrophe or find new ways to deal with a problem, ensure you reach out for support. Be kind to yourself— even recognising a fixed or negative mindset is a positive step forward.

Social interaction can be hugely beneficial to help you deal with challenges, such as venting about a situation or getting help to find new possibilities which you may not see for yourself. Whether you are dealing with a severe medical issue, an injury, a personal challenge like financial or family problems, overwhelm, or fear of getting started on your fitness journey, dig out the list of support people from your toolbox, and reach out for help.

I know that having patience, realistic expectations, self-compassion, gratitude for our bodies and the right support, will lead us to take those small steps to get back on track. Expressing and sharing our concerns out loud, rather than keeping them bottled up inside, can stop us from a feeling a sense of hopelessness, can lighten our mood and help shift our viewpoint.

Working with clients who have physical and mental challenges has enriched my life and taught me valuable lessons in compassion and gratitude. I feel inspired by their resilience and positive attitudes to focus on their CAN-DO approach and their receptiveness to try new things, even in the face of adversity.

Some of the challenges that prevent us from exercising:
- busy lives with limited time
- physical injuries or limitations, medical conditions
- difficult circumstances involving finances, family situation, isolation, transport
- mental or psychological issues ranging from negative mindset and confidence through to severe problems that can include grief, sadness, loneliness and depression.

The ways we deal with individual challenges will be varied; however, I have shared some ideas below. I invite you to take on board any that may be useful for you and encourage you to practise them with patience and baby steps.

If you are working with a health professional, then ensure you give them ALL the information, so they can assist you with the best strategies and liaise with other people on your team. By recognising when your mindset or other issue is affecting your motivation to exercise, you will be better equipped to find solutions.

'Courage doesn't always roar. Sometimes courage is the quiet voice at the end of the day saying, "I will try again tomorrow".'
– Mary Anne Radmacher

1. BE YOUR OWN BEST BUDDY!

Have you ever had an injury or not received the expected quick results and paid out on yourself? I hear people at the gym referring to their bodies in a negative way quite often. Our individual challenges can be small and varied but big in our own minds.

I once heard Deepak Chopra talk about dealing with challenges on his *Perfect Health Meditation* series podcast. He said, '*There are likely some days when it is challenging to send positive messages to the body. Maybe you are living with a difficult illness or you feel tired all the time, or your clothes fit too tightly—when we perceive that our bodies have aged, are unfit, weak or diseased we tend to focus on what we believe is wrong. We tell ourselves "I don't like you".*

Imagine though, that this ache, sickness or condition was a friend sitting right before you sad and weeping. We wouldn't ignore her or express irritation. Instead we would embrace her and nurture her offering her words of encouragement and love. It's the same for our bodies. When we have an ache, pain, sickness or perceived imperfection, it is important that we acknowledge those areas and offer them love and acceptance.'

I reflect on those wise words often to practise positive self-talk and feel gratitude for my own body. Deepak Chopra also said:

'Our body is the vehicle to take us on the journey of life. Our body is worthy of the best of our care. The body reflects back to us what we offer it. Our bodies take care of us responding to feedback loops we create that are integral to health and wellbeing. Positive self-talk nurtures every cell, muscle and organ and supports health and vitality.'

If you have an issue that is preventing you from being more physically active:

- don't compare yourself with others
- accept your limitation without defeatism or 'if only' thinking
- trust yourself to know your own body best, know when to push and encourage, when to back off
- others can't possibly know what it's like to be in your shoes so keep this in mind when dealing with other people too
- do what is possible for you, even if you can't do your regular activity—any is better than none
- on challenging days when movement is hard, be kind to yourself and look ahead to a new day
- be patient and flexible if you can't start or resume an activity that you previously enjoyed. Adopt a questioning mindset to explore **what CAN I do?**
- if you can't move, use your time in a productive way—research ideas for the future of how you will transition to a different way of moving
- practise meditation, conscious breathing and mindfulness techniques. Keeping perspective when faced with an obstacle can be easier with a clear mind, and it will also help you manage negative stress
- stay connected with friends, family and professionals to help get you moving. It can also help to talk to others that have been down the same path, in an online group or in person

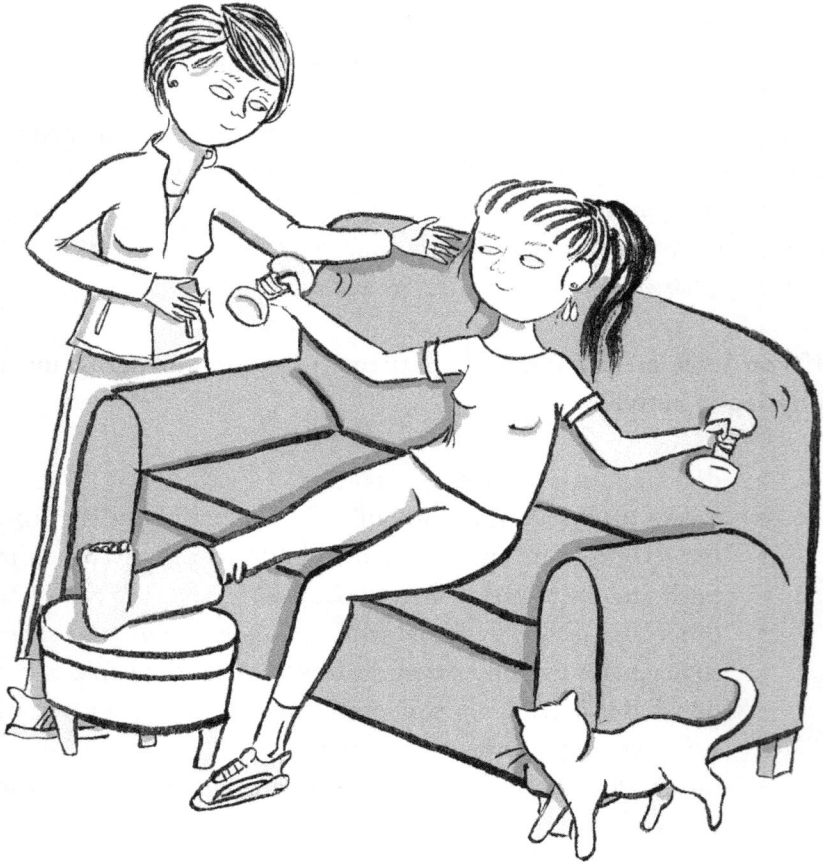

- accept offers of help. It might be you need to talk about something that is worrying you, or you might need the opposite—to focus on something unrelated
- distraction with humour can be a great medicine!

2. PROBLEM SOLVING

Advance planning

If you 'play it by ear' and wait to see how you feel in the morning, exercise may not happen. Advance planning will help you stay committed.

This strategy worked well for Dana, who suffered from an autoimmune disorder, obesity and depression. She struggled to get out of bed and be motivated enough to do any form of exercise.

Dana booked a block of twice-weekly personal training sessions to motivate her to get out of bed and move. If she did not have the sessions pre-booked, she was at risk of staying in bed until lunchtime. Dana valued keeping her word and didn't want to let me down by not showing up, so pre-booking became her winning strategy. It would still be a struggle to get out of bed, but the thought of letting someone down, allowed her to push through her mental barriers. As a bonus, she enjoyed the exercise and experienced many positive benefits.

I'm not suggesting that this is the answer for everyone with issues like depression, although it could be worth trying such a strategy with the support of an understanding health professional.

'On the other side of a storm is the strength that comes from having navigated through it. Raise your sail and begin.'
– Gregory S Williams

Recognise your foggy filter

When we feel overwhelmed and in a negative mindset, we can view life through a foggy filter, and it can be hard to find solutions. Excuses can become a barrier, and the desire to navigate our way out can be lost.

If we can be consciously aware when we are seeing things in a distorted or negative way, we can reach out for help or problem solve when feeling better.

One of my clients, Jackie, 51, recognised that she was carrying around 'but what if' excuses in her head and couldn't see clearly enough to find the answers. Asking for help was the first step, and together we problem solved to overcome her resistance to getting to the gym.

Jackie was overweight and at high risk for heart disease. She had been medically prescribed exercise and modifications to her diet. Jackie was battling with hormonal issues and experienced severe hot flushes, insomnia and mood swings. She worried about how she might cope with the discomfort and embarrassment of hot flushes during exercise. Besides that, after a restless sleep, she felt too tired to exercise. Her strategy so far, had been to complain and stay home by the cool air conditioner and justify why she could not exercise. This was getting her nowhere and was contributing to her moodiness at home.

Jackie's daughter brought her to see me, frustrated by her mum's defeatist attitude. After validating her concerns, we reached a solution. Jackie agreed to a six-week trial of personal training sessions and committed to turn up to ALL sessions regardless of how tired or miserable she felt (unless she was sick). In return, I would not be forcing her to skip and jump as she had been visualising in her head! I would incorporate frequent breaks and modify the intensity and style of exercise to suit her on that particular day, even if that meant lying on a foam roller doing mobility and breathwork. Indoor or outdoor training would be determined by the weather.

We also diarised appropriate group fitness classes including aqua classes (water can be very therapeutic). To assist with accountability, we paired Jackie up with a training buddy, with her daughter as a 'reserve'. Jackie could work at her own pace with a lower impact if necessary.

By taking small steps to build confidence, this approach paid off. I've now trained Jackie for several years and we often laugh about her preconceived ideas of what she thought I would make her do!

Putting such strategies in place can relieve a lot of mental anguish over the perception of scenarios that may never even happen. In Jackie's case, for her to know that she had people on her side, not forcing but encouraging, helped transition her into developing confidence and stepping out of her comfort zone. Once she started to notice small wins (like how exercise was becoming easier) and was reaping some tangible benefits, it became easier for her to continue.

I have encountered many 'Jackies' including people with shyness or embarrassment about a weight issue who preferred to hide in the corner. Just know that if you ever have a *Jackie* moment, there are always solutions, even if the fog is preventing you from seeing them. Ensure you divulge all reservations, even if you think you are the only person to ever feel that way. Chances are, you are not.

If you are problem-solving an issue on your own, try writing down all the possible solutions as if you were advising a friend. For example: '**What if** I wake up with a sore back and can't go to pump class? **Then I will** go for a swim in the pool'. '**What if** I don't feel motivated to go walking? **Then I will** ask a friend to join me.'

3. A MATTER OF TIME ...

'I don't have enough time!' Take the phrase out of your vocab or rephrase it! Remember, the question is not about finding more time; it is about your priorities. Here are a few more tips:

Plan for it!
- Plan your diary for the week ahead. Block out three or four planned exercise sessions and make appointments with *yourself* to build a regular routine of *some* exercise *every* day, even for 10-minute blocks. Keep the commitment going and celebrate ticking those achievements off! When unexpected challenges arise, ramp up as much incidental activity as possible.

- Keep it interesting and varied with new classes, walking or swimming dates with friends, book in (and pre-pay) for lessons to learn a new skill, or explore a new neighbourhood or park. It is a bonus to enjoy what you are doing and who you are doing it with!

- Challenge your, 'I'm not a morning person' inner dialogue to find out if it is true. Lay out your morning clothes, set your alarm (out of reach) and get to bed early. Give it a try more than once! Then you can decide.

- Change up your usual routine and incorporate a pre- or post-dinner workout or walk, even if it is only for five minutes. You can build up the time gradually. Record it in your diary and add on an extra minute or more each day.

- Push back on yourself and reassess your priorities next time you say, 'I don't have time to exercise'. Consider social media habits and use timers to keep in check.

Be organised!

If you ARE ultra-busy with limited time, ensure you are not wasting time by having a cluttered environment. Clutter can have negative effects on your mental and physical health.

- Try devoting an entire weekend to decluttering and organising your whole house for a fresh start, not just the pantry and fridge. Use a timer to stay focused, working your way through one complete room before going to the next. If you live with others, enrol them in the idea (with enticements if necessary). Block out a date, schedule it in your diary and get serious about it. You might even engage a professional cleaner to help.

- On a separate weekend, declutter your computer and inbox. Re-organise your clothing too.

- When you are decluttering, put your phone on silent and have a digital detox for a whole day or two. If you absolutely can't manage without checking out your Instagram or Facebook feed, set a timer for 10 minutes at the end of the day for a tiny SM fix.

You will feel so clear-headed after decluttering and be re-energised for a fresh start. Try introducing some new daily or weekly actions to keep your environment clear.

Q&A

Q. How do I modify my exercise when injured?

Get good advice from a medical or fitness professional. Be open-minded to try alternative activities that are safe for you. Be patient.

Q. I'm feeling isolated and lacking in motivation to exercise.

Your support team can be a great resource to you right now. Engage socially as much as possible, even online, or engage a coach or trainer to help you vent your feelings and assist with a plan.

Q. What if I'm injured and can't exercise or prepare my usual healthy food?

Aim to be solution-focused and look for answers, not problems. Ask for help to brainstorm ideas to help you through this phase to move forward in a positive way.

IN A NUTSHELL:

- **We have a choice** how we view obstacles. Adopt a growth mindset and look for opportunities. Find your silver linings.

- **Focus on what you CAN do**, not what you CAN'T. Don't give up!

- **Cultivate an 'own best friend' belief**, feel gratitude and compassion for your own body.

- **Practise meditation** and mindfulness techniques.

- **Problem-solve with advance planning**. Ask for help and seek social support.

- **Plan for 'what if' problems** with 'then I will' solutions and write them down.

- **Challenge your 'I don't have time' beliefs** and make healthy habits a priority.

- **Declutter** your environment.

CHAPTER 12

Your Inner Spark
Loving the new, healthier you

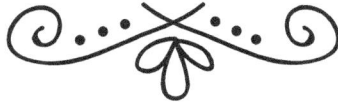

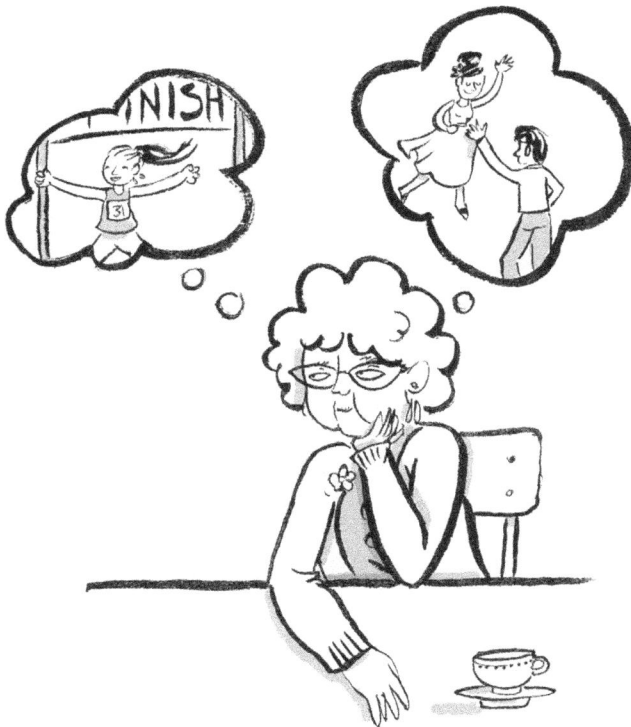

'Twenty years from now, you will be more disappointed by the things that you didn't do than by the ones you did do. So, throw off the bowlines. Catch the trade winds in your sails. Explore. Dream. Discover.'

– Mark Twain

It is my wish that you will have generated excitement and a fresh outlook towards your health and fitness and can be proud to celebrate your commitment to reclaim your optimal wellness with new vigour and passion.

Wellness is an ongoing journey. Some days we can feel on top of the world, rocketing along at full speed, blitzing and ticking off things left, right and centre. Not every day will be perfect, and that is reality and doesn't mean we have failed. There is learning to be gained in every situation, even if we don't see it at that very moment—it sometimes shows up on reflection, *if* we are open to seeing it.

Be consistent and keep going with your new set of actions, even on those days when you might not feel like it, by modifying plans as required. YOU make the rules; this is YOUR journey. Perfectionism can bring pressure and obsessive stress, so don't view wellness as if it is an end goal to reach like a type of enlightenment at the top of the mountain. It really is the *everyday* part of the journey and how we view it that brings inner joy and happiness.

Whilst you will have goals that have a definite end point, allow your vision to expand and evolve as you change and grow. Ensure your vision continues to generate excitement and a desire to keep learning and growing to be living the best life possible. Review it often and see your vision as that wonderful bright, dazzling light to show you the way and propel you into action, bringing meaning to your actions and goals.

It's okay to change course

Celebrate your wins along the way. Did you set out to achieve one thing but changed course as priorities shifted? Be flexible.

Reflecting back on my fitness journey almost 15 years ago, I started for health and weight loss reasons but what I got out of it, far exceeded my expectations. As someone that had previously considered formal exercise a chore, I discovered joy and confidence and new opportunities to share my passion for good health.

Keep learning

Just as we are nourished by healthy food and exercise, the process of **learning** nourishes our minds and keeps us open to new opportunities and experiences. We can feel invigorated after listening to an inspiring TED talk or gain a fresh perspective from an interesting book.

My inner spark has ignited a thirst for knowledge and keeps me on my toes. Stepping into uncomfortable and raising the bar to try new challenges, is scary and exciting. Studying new science and writing this book has me feeling this way!

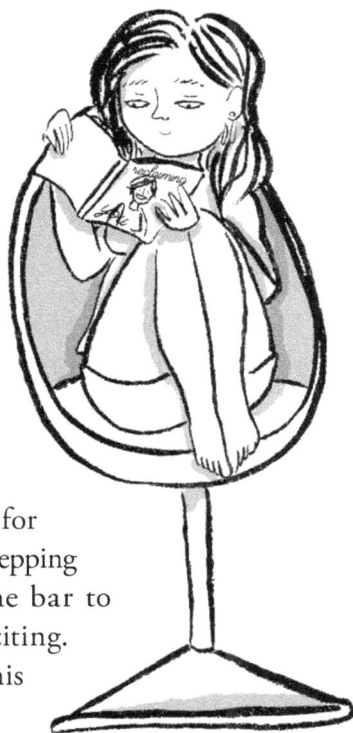

Your first steps

If you don't feel ready to step onto the path and start your new journey, ask yourself, what *would* it take for you to commence making changes to your health? What are you waiting for? Only you can decide but don't leave it too long or wait until all the stars are lined up to begin. Take those first steps.

Hopefully you *are* motivated to begin although sometimes, it can be hard just to kick off. Initiating action is far harder than sustaining it so I suggest that you don't wait for tomorrow—get started NOW! Here are some final tips to ensure this happens:

Daily action plan: Write down three easy tasks that you can achieve today. It could be as simple as making enquiries about a class, trying a new healthy drink, going shopping for workout clothes or shoes, two minutes of conscious breathing or reading an article that makes you laugh or smile. Make it happen!

Revise: Go back to each chapter and use the 'In a Nutshell' as a prompt to remind you of strategies to try or re-read a chapter as required.

Plan for your ideal day: Consider some new routines to incorporate into your ideal day and introduce changes gradually. This might include an **early morning** or **bedtime routine** that could include a few minutes of gentle stretching, reading, pampering or a stroll around the garden to greet the new day or check out the beautiful night sky.

Becoming an early riser and having a morning routine allows me to have more 'me' time before the rest of the household is awake, and it sets me up well for the day. No demands, no rushing, such a peaceful time of day with freedom to choose whatever I feel like doing. Technology and newsfeeds can wait! I also enjoy an evening ritual that includes a few minutes of stargazing and time for reflection and gratitude for the wonder of my life.

Celebrate: Making good choices will become easier each day and before long, you will default to the best choice in auto mode with ease. Celebrate and be proud of your daily success!

Writing has given me an exciting opportunity to revisit my own journey and share it with you. After reading this book, I hope you too can feel that inner spark and a desire to keep learning to bring more movement, joy, wellness and happiness into your life.

Create your vision, find your inner spark and go for it.

Enjoy Reclaiming You!

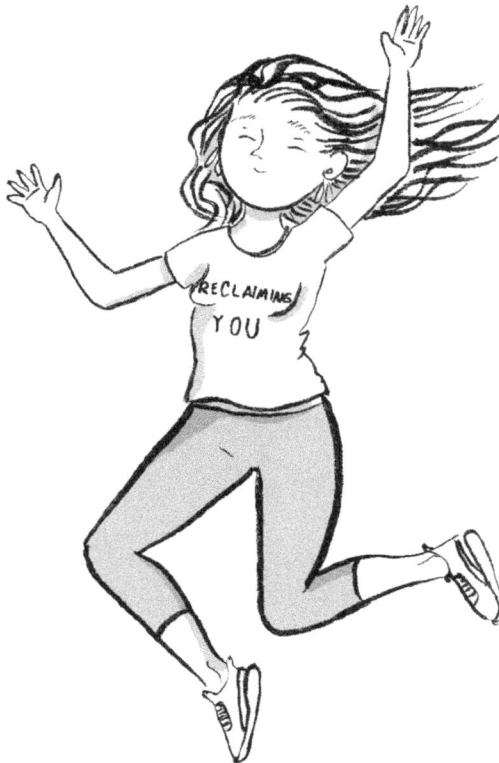

Afterword

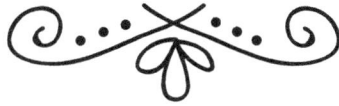

When writing this book, it was challenging to put down on paper what I cover in live coaching sessions.

Those sessions are not scripted to follow an exact 'dot point' process as set out in this book, and I adapt methods to suit the individual and circumstances at that time.

Our learning styles and preferences are also unique—once again, one size does not fit all!

There are many ways to explore and create visions and goals that are effective. If the structured method of instructions contained in this book does not suit your style, then adapt it for your own needs. If you would like to have some additional help and work with me further, please contact me to discuss options. Individual coaching can be arranged.

- Want to stay in touch and be the first to know about my upcoming wellness workshops and events?

- Like to find out more about getting a personalised health assessment and program and hear more about epigenetics?

Please subscribe to the link on my website for updates.

Thank you so much for reading this book. If you have any feedback, queries or success stories to share, then drop me a line on my email address below. I would love to hear from you.

I wish you all the very best for your future health and trust you will enjoy your wellness journey.

Jeanette

www.reclaimingyou.com.au

jeanette@reclaimingyou.com.au

About The Author

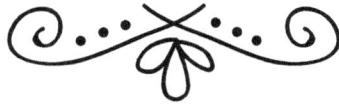

Jeanette Herrington is a highly regarded, energetic personal trainer and health coach from Perth, Western Australia. She is dedicated and passionate about helping newcomers to gain confidence and joy around fitness.

Jeanette was born and raised in Yarrawonga, a beautiful country town in Victoria. At 21, she left her hometown, embarked on a working holiday and settled in Perth several years later.

Having experienced her own challenge to regain fitness after having children in her 40s, Jeanette succeeded in getting back on track and developed a newfound love of exercise and living a healthy lifestyle. This led to her embarking on a new career in the health and fitness industry, to inspire other women like her, and she has now been a successful fitness professional for over a decade.

A varied and adventurous working background has helped Jeanette relate to clients from all walks of life. With many years of experience working in law firms, crewing on a yacht in the South Pacific and stints in hospitality, including managing a world famous 5-star Fijian resort, her interesting past brings forward a fresh future.

Jeanette is currently presenting wellness sessions for 'Roll Back the Clock' program, a Bowls Australia initiative to assist senior Australians 'find their 30'. Her book, *Reclaiming You* aims to motivate other women to take those first steps to have a healthier lifestyle, with exercise as a lifelong partner.

When Jeanette is not training clients, she loves family time out and about in nature and aspires to be a healthy role model to her two teenage daughters.

Jeanette can be contacted via the link on her website at **www.reclaimingyou.com.au.**

Acknowledgements

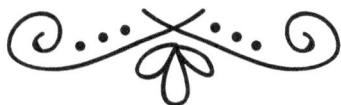

What an adventure I've had creating this book, one that has sparked excitement in me to jump out of bed and get writing, even sometimes sacrificing my early morning walk! The writing journey has been challenging and at the same time invigorating as I've raced against the clock to finish this before my next big birthday!

Whilst writing this book, I realised how much my upbringing has influenced my journey and ideas I've shared. I acknowledge my parents, Pamela and Malcolm and my beautiful sister Susan, for the solid grounding I've had. I'm so grateful to you for a happy start to life with ongoing love and support, and for instilling good values in me along with important life skills.

Reflecting further on those skills, I've recognised how resilience and a positive attitude has helped me to complete this book. Mum, you have always encouraged me to never give up and adapt plans to keep going. In my younger days, you helped me to adjust plans when I was tempted to quit! I will continue to be inspired by the resilience, wisdom and positivity that you both have shared. Dad, you lived a wonderful life into your 90s with strength and determination. You always encouraged me to pursue my purpose in life and to see things through to completion. Even now, it's still appropriate with your recent passing and doesn't diminish anything. I'll miss you so much my darling dad and will reflect on your wise words often.

Thank you to my gorgeous, caring daughters, Charlize and Amberley. I appreciate your love, support, patience and the practical help you've given me whilst I wrote this book, especially when I lost track of time, complained about deadlines and forgot all about dinner and had to fall back on toasted sandwiches. Lucky I always had soup on tap and a budding young master chef in the family! Peter, you've been so encouraging and supportive of my writing and a valuable sounding board too. I truly appreciate your time and expert help with tech issues and for taking the cover photo as well. Your generosity to ensure I had all the tools of the trade, including a brand-new computer, made writing this book much easier! *Vinaka vakalevu!* Thank you also to my young at heart, mother-in-law Dorothy, for your enthusiastic support and understanding, particularly when I had to cancel our visits so I could meet deadlines!

Thanks to all my friends for their encouragement and good company. Just know that I'm back in circulation and ready for *walk n talk* any time! For my work colleague and good friend Barb, thank you for your enthusiastic and valuable contribution. It is truly appreciated and I've loved sharing SK writing stories with you! I particularly want to acknowledge my dearest friend and confidante Lindy. You top me up with positive support on a daily basis with your inspirational text messages filled with friendly hearts and emojis, cheering me on to complete my book. Everyone needs a 'Lindy' in their lives—to use her words, 'can you be cloned'?

My clients, past and present, thank you for entrusting me to be your training coach and for sharing so generously with me. In particular, I want to acknowledge Vanessa. Even on challenging days, you turn up to training no matter what and inspire me with your positive attitude, willing to give anything a go.

Special thanks to Natasa and Stuart Denman, Vivienne Mason, Julie Fisher, Lendy Macario and the team at Ultimate World Publishing for your belief in me and for your generous help, guidance and reassurance.

Thanks to Pamela Carrington for the fabulous illustrations, book cover designer, Nikola Boskovski and my editor Marinda Wilkinson for their valuable input and support as well as my new author buddies. I feel so fortunate to have you all on my team!

Thank you to my personal support team of health and fitness professionals that have kept me accountable, energised and moving well despite many hours sitting at a computer writing this book. I appreciate all of your care, personalised attention and generosity to share information. To Dr Cam McDonald and all the presenters of workshops, seminars, classes and other professionals and friends in the fitness industry, I acknowledge and appreciate you all for the way you have helped to shape my thoughts and consolidate my learning.

Finally, to you the reader, thank you for reading my book on wellness. I also appreciate those who pre-ordered it and have waited so patiently. Enjoy!

Event Speaker

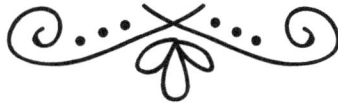

Jeanette is an enthusiastic presenter and author. She loves to share her passion for wellness, particularly with women who want to improve their health. Her book, *Reclaiming You* aims to motivate women to take those first steps to making lasting positive changes to feel energised and confident.

A varied and adventurous working background has helped Jeanette relate to clients from all walks of life. Prior to becoming a fitness professional 12 years ago, she had many years of experience working in law firms, crewing on a yacht in the South Pacific and stints in hospitality, including managing a world famous 5-star Fijian resort.

Jeanette is a highly regarded personal trainer and health coach and is currently presenting wellness sessions for Bowls Australia, as part of their 'Roll back the Clock' Program.

If you would like Jeanette to tailor a wellness presentation to suit your audience, please contact her for more details.

www.reclaimingyou.com.au
jeanette@reclaimingyou.com.au

References

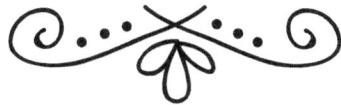

Andrei, Mihai 2018, *What calories look like in different foods*, ZME Science, viewed 20 September 2020, < https://www.zmescience.com/other/feature-post/calories-different-foods/>.

Australian Institute of Health and Welfare 2020, *Deaths in Australia*, Australian Institute of Health and Welfare, viewed 20 September 2020, <https://www.aihw.gov.au/reports/life-expectancy-death/deaths-in-australia/contents/leading-causes-of-death>.

Australian Fitness Network, 2019 online course *Coaching Skills for Maximal Client Results* incorporating presentations by Dr Cam McDonald.

Burns, Stephanie 1993, *Great Lies We Live By*, Caminole Pty Limited Australia

Burns, Stephanie 2020, Stephanie Burns, website, viewed 17 October 2020, <https://www.stephanieburns.com/materials/articles>.

Chopra, Deepak 2020, Deepak Chopra, website, viewed 20 September 2020, <https://www.chopra.com>.

Chopra, Deepak 2013, *Perfect health 21-Day meditation challenge*, viewed 20 September 2020, <https://chopracentermeditation.com/store/product/2/perfect_health_streaming>.

Clear, James 2018, *Atomic habits: an easy and proven way to build good habits and break bad ones*, Cornerstone, London.

Coyle, Daniel 2010, *The talent code: greatness isn't born, it's grown*, Cornerstone, London.

Duhigg, Charles 2020, How habits work, Charles Duhigg, viewed 20 September 2020, < https://www.charlesduhigg.com/how-habits-work/>.

Dweck, Carol 2017, *Mindset: changing the way you think to fulfil your potential*, updated edition, Little Brown Book Group, London.

Eady, Julie 2017, *Additive alert: your guide to safer shopping*, 3rd edition, Woodslane, Sydney.

Enders, Giulia 2015, *Gut: The inside story of our body's most under-rated organ*, Scribe, Melbourne.

Fitness Australia 2020, website, viewed 20 September 2020, <https://www.fitness.org.au>.

Fleming, Jennifer & Bouvier, Anna-Louise 2010, *The feel good body: 7 steps to easing aches and looking great*, HarperCollins Publishers, Sydney.

Fuller, Andrew 2016, *'Brain-based learning for parents workshop'*, Perth <https://www.andrewfuller.com.au>.

Gameau, Damon & Zoe 2016, *That Sugar Guide: practical tips to get you eating real foods again*, Pan Macmillan, Melbourne.

Health Direct 2020, *Essential screening tests for men*, Health Direct, viewed 20 September 2020, <https://www.healthdirect.gov.au/essential-screening-tests-for-men>.

Health Direct 2020, *Health checks for women*, Health Direct, viewed 20 September 2020, <https://www.healthdirect.gov.au/health-checks-for-women>.

Heart Foundation of Australia 2020, *Key statistics: Heart disease in Australia*, Heart Foundation of Australia, viewed 20 September 2020, <https://www.heartfoundation.org.au/About-us/Australia-Heart-Disease-Statistics>.

Intuitive Eating 2019, 10 principals of intuitive eating, blog article, viewed 17 October 2020, <https://www.intuitiveeating.org/10-principles-of-intuitive-eating/>.

McDonald, Dr Cam, *The ultimate in behaviour change seminar for health professionals*, presented at Filex, Sydney, viewed online 2019, <https://www.fitnessnetwork.com.au/>.

Northrup, Dr Christiane 2009, *The wisdom of menopause*, Little Brown Book Group, London.

Positive Psychology 2020, website, viewed 17 October 2020, <https://www.positivepsychology.com/category/gratitude/>.

Ratey, John J 2013, *Spark: The revolutionary new science of exercise and the brain,* reprint edition, Little Brown and Company, New York.

That Sugar Film 2014, motion picture, Madman Entertainment, Melbourne.

Williams, Bri 2018, *The how of habits*, Bri Williams, Melbourne.

Notes

Notes

Notes

www.ingramcontent.com/pod-product-compliance
Lightning Source LLC
Chambersburg PA
CBHW032054020426
42335CB00011B/339